HELP WITH THE NURSING PROCESS

A MANAGEMENT GUIDE

by

Davina J. Gosnell, R.N., Ph.D.

ANOTHER

HEALTHCARE AGENCY
EDUCATIONAL AND
LEARNING
PROGRAM

FOR THE BENEFIT OF

- *Your Patients or Clients*
- *Your Coworkers*
- *Your Employer*
- *Yourself*

HELP #19 in the Management Guide Series

Publishers

W.L. Ganong Company, Healthcare Management Consultants
P.O. Box 2727, Chapel Hill, North Carolina 27514

Publishers:
W. L. Ganong Company, P.O. Box 2727
Chapel Hill, North Carolina 27514

Library of Congress Catalog Card Number: 80-66120
ISBN: 0-933036-19-1

2 3 4 5

C O N T E N T S

Davina Gosnell is a nurse consultant associate with the W.L. Ganong
Company, Healthcare Management Consultants. She has a broad background as a nurse consultant, manager and educator.

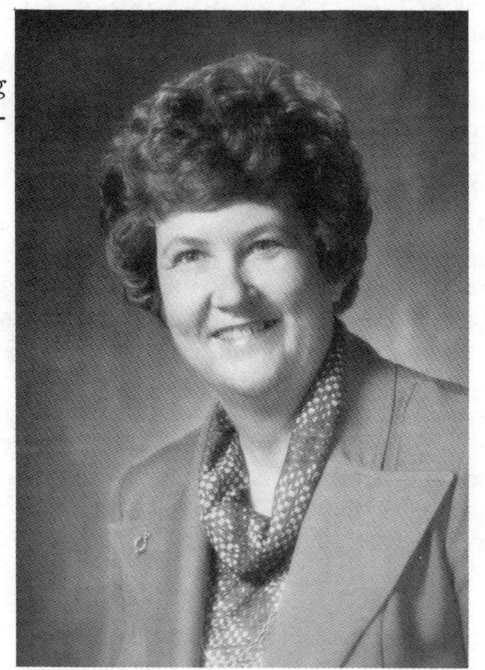

Dr. Gosnell earned her Ph.D. in
Adult Education at The Ohio State
University after having first re-
ceived her diploma in nursing at
Massillon City Hospital School of
Nursing in Massillon, Ohio; her
BS in Nursing at the University
of Pittsburgh; and her MS at The
Ohio State University.

During those years she progressed
from staff nurse and team leader
at Massillon City Hospital and
the University of Pittsburgh Stu-
dent Health Service to faculty
member at Presbyterian-University
Hospital School of Nursing. For
seven years she was a supervisor and then nursing consultant in
home health services at the Ohio Department of Health. Her responsibilities included work with agency personnel regarding
nursing practice, and nursing management consultation with administrative and supervisory staffs of home health agencies.

Dr. Gosnell serves as an associate professor of nursing at Kent
State University. She is a member of Sigma Theta Tau, and active
professionally in a wide variety of nursing and educational associations.

FOREWORD

The nursing process is a systematic problem-solving approach
to nursing that provides for the delivery of nursing care
most appropriate to each patient's specific needs and problems. It gives nurses a structure by which to better organize, coordinate and deliver nursing care. Communication and
evaluation are keystones. Assessment, planning, implementation, and evaluation are the four major steps of the cyclical
process. The nursing process is applicable in any nursing
setting and with any client/patient.

The purpose of this manual is to assist nurses who want to
enhance nursing practice and provide excellence in patient
care. Much has been written about the nursing process.
Within the realm of practice, however, we see somewhat
limited use made of the concepts and principles of the
nursing process. Often we find bits and pieces of the process being used; but it is the exception to find a well-
coordinated program of nursing care delivery in which all
phases of the process are consistently carried out in a syn-
chronized fashion.

This manual is designed to help you, the nurse, utilize the
nursing process with your patients in the clinical setting
where you work. Upon completion of this course of study,
you—the learner—should be better able to:

1. Explain each step of the nursing process.

2. Conduct nursing assessments.

3. Develop comprehensive patient care plans.

4. Implement nursing care based upon assessment
   and planning.

5. Identify and utilize evaluation techniques to
   determine the adequacy, appropriateness, efficiency, and effectiveness of nursing care
   provided.

6. Document each step of the nursing process.

May you enjoy learning to provide better patient care. My
thanks to one and all who assisted, either directly or indirectly, in the preparation of this manual.

Kent, Ohio   Davina J. Gosnell
January, 1980

<u>Response Sheet No. 1</u>

SELF-ADMINISTERED PRE-TEST

<u>Instructions</u>: Please list what you <u>know</u> and how you <u>feel</u> about this subject (before beginning your study program). Include as many items as possible, briefly and frankly. Use other side if necessary.

FACTS (Cognitive Information): What I <u>Know</u> About This Subject	FEELINGS (Affective Information): How I <u>Feel</u> About This Subject
	Identify your feelings about each fact.
1.	1. Some <u>Feelings</u> *Agitated* *Amused*
2.	2. *Angry* *Anxious* *Apprehensive* *Belittled*
3.	3. *Bemused* *Bewildered* *Confused* *Content*
4.	4. *Depressed* *Disaffected* *Excited* *Expectant*
5.	5. *Faint* *Foolish* *Glad* *Happy*
6.	6. *Hurt* *Impressed* *Inspired* *Irritated*
7.	7. *Joyful* *Kindly* *Lost* *Morose*
8.	8. *Numb* *Optimistic* *Proud* *Provoked*
9.	9. *Puzzled* *Queer* *Querulous* *Relieved*
10.	10. *Sorrowful* *Stunned* *Thrilled* *Upset* *Wondering*

NAME _________________________________ TITLE _________________________________ DATE

AGENCY _______________________________ CITY & ZIP ____________________________

HELP WITH UNDERSTANDING THE NURSING PROCESS

*Individualized, goal-directed nursing care
shall be provided to patients through the
use of the nursing process.*

Nursing Services Standard IV, JCAH
Accreditation Manual for Hospitals, 1980

Conceptual Framework

Nursing process is one of the simplest yet most complex concepts ever introduced in nursing. The structural model of Figure 1 is fairly simple, showing the basic elements as a four-step cyclical process.

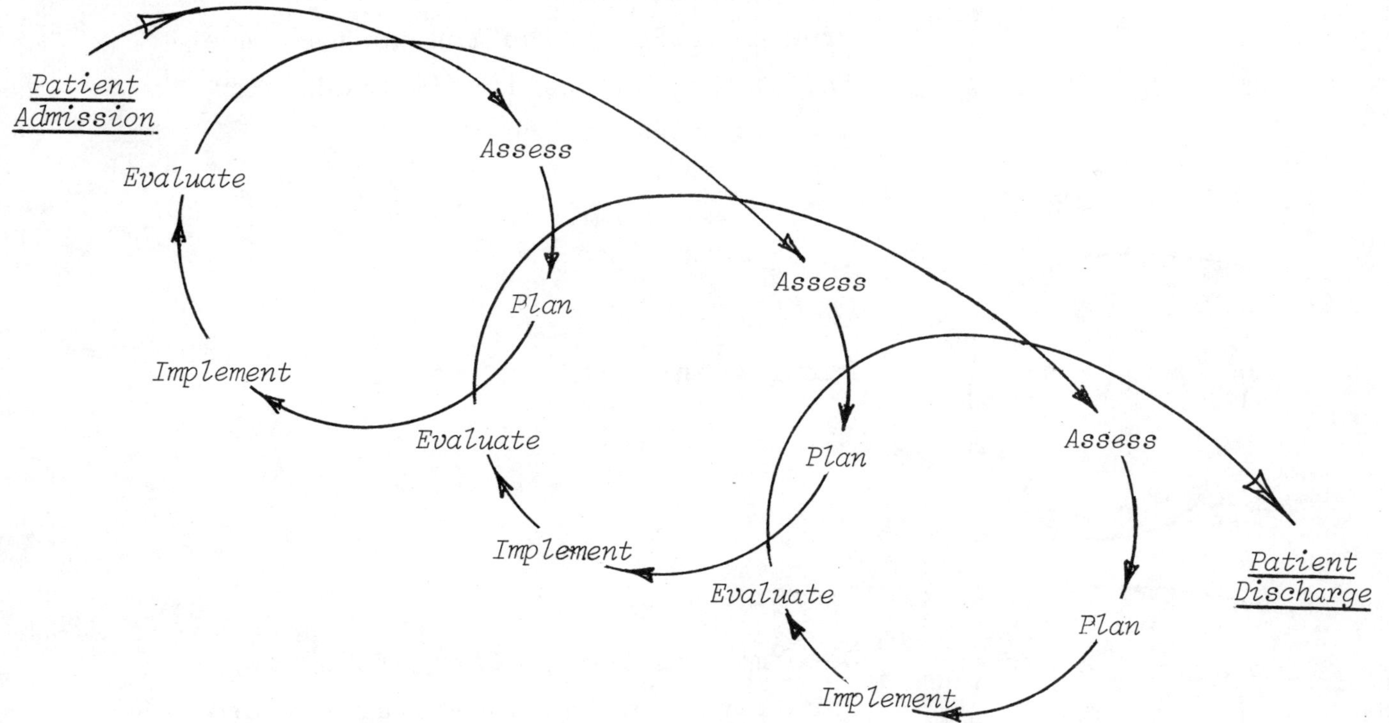

THE NURSING PROCESS CYCLE

Figure 1

Definitions

The nursing process is based upon scientific problem-solving, a most relevant and utilitarian model. The four steps are assessing, planning, implementing, and evaluating. Whenever possible, the patient must participate directly in each of these steps. The patient is the focus of the process.

ASSESS: Size up the patient.

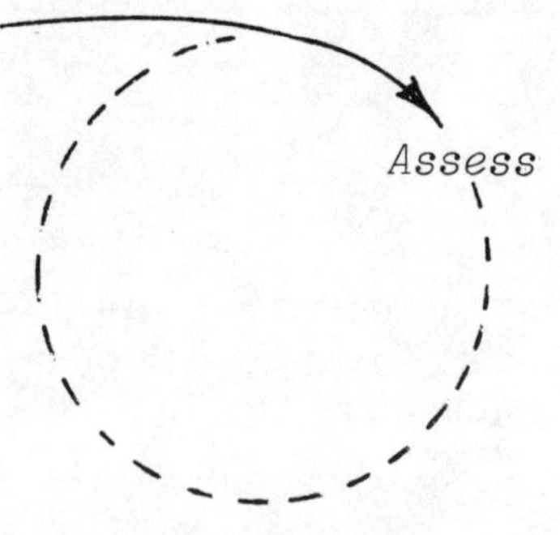

Systematic gathering of information about a patient's health and illness, then analyzing the information using nursing knowledge and judgment to determine individual patient problems and needs for nursing care.

PLAN: Decide what to do.

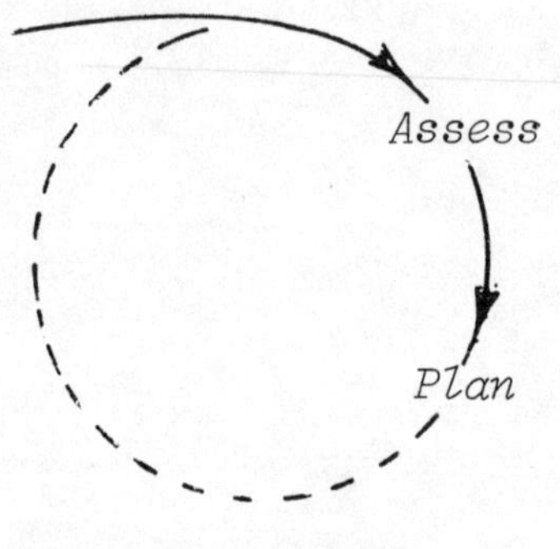

Formulating nursing activities in order to accomplish the goal of meeting individual patient's needs for nursing care.

IMPLEMENT: Do it.

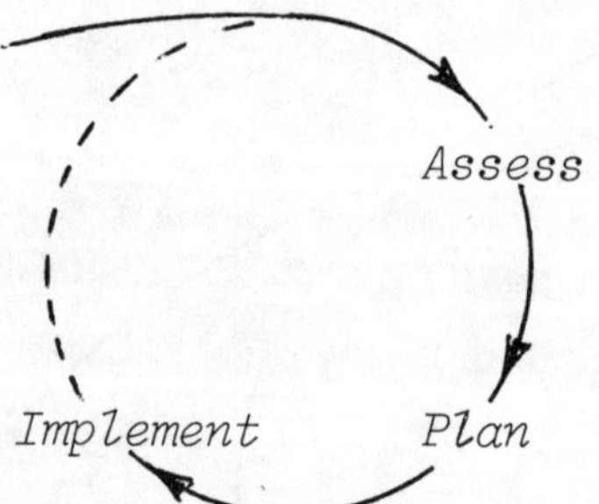

Putting into effect the plan of care.

EVALUATE: Did it work?

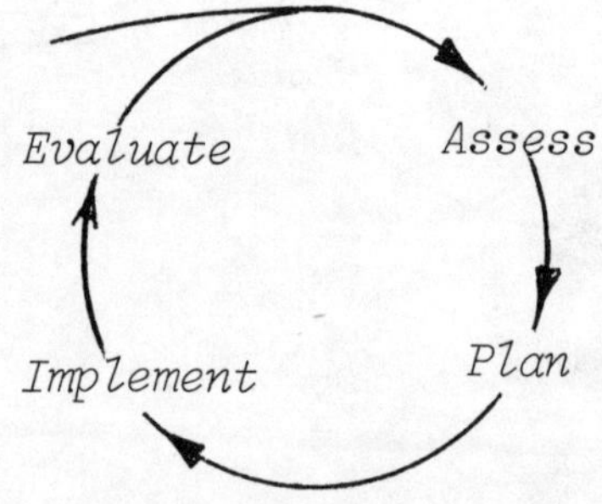

Determining the quality of nursing care provided and assessing the progress of the patient in attaining health goals.

Process is defined as a series of actions, changes or functions that bring about a particular result. The *result* is the nursing care that is individualized to the needs of each patient. Nursing process is a method by which nursing is practiced. It is utilitarian; it can be used by all nurses regardless of the settings in which they practice or the nursing needs of the patient/client.

Why Nursing Process

The nursing profession has a rich heritage. Although the era of modern nursing began with Nightingale in the mid-19th century, nursing's origin is prehistoric, for within every civilization there have been persons designated to attend and comfort the sick.

Nightingale's modern nursing era brought with it more formalized nursing education and the establishment of initial standards of expected nursing practice. Although Nightingale did not describe nursing process, she did note factors that today are recognized as part of the nursing process. For example,

> *If you cannot get in the habit of*
> *observation one way or another, you*
> *had better give up being a nurse.*
> Nightingale, Notes on Nursing

Later in this manual we will address the important role observation has in assessment, the first step of nursing process.

Rapid changes in health care and nursing have come in the 20th century. In the early 1900's the majority of medical care was provided by the general practitioner and most nurses were employed in a private duty role. Only persons gravely ill were confined to the hospital. By mid-century it was common to have health insurance, hospitals were being built in nearly every community with Hill-Burton funds and the public was learning to view the hospital as the core of health-care delivery. Physician specialization was common, and greater numbers of nurses than ever before were being graduated.

In the decades since, medical technology has provided highly complex equipment which allows for monitoring, life support, dialysis and organ transplants. Laboratory studies, diagnostic

procedures, surgical interventions and medical management
are highly specialized. Healthcare is recognized as the
second or third largest industry in the country. In addition
to the nurse and physician, a large number of different health
workers have been added, including therapists, social workers,
and numerous non-professional technicians and aides, who are
now regarded as part of the health care team.

The health care delivery system today represents complexity
of the highest order. Change is endemic. Innovative concepts
are being introduced constantly in response to increased demand for health services, the improvement of consumer access,
better utilization of available manpower and facilities, and
the control of spiraling costs. Preventive screening programs,
ambulatory centers, day care, health maintenance organizations
(HMOs), wholistic health centers, and hospices are some
examples.

Nursing throughout this modern era has faced challenge and
change. "What is nursing?" is a question that has been asked
repeatedly. An examination of the sociological characteristics of nurses and their roles and functions was the focus of
the majority of early studies. Findings revealed great vari-
ances in practice and no unifying framework by which to char-
acterize nursing. Nursing activities were rapidly changing,
as many of the traditional nursing tasks were assumed by new
health workers, and physicians were delegating to nurses more
and more duties previously performed exclusively by the doctor.

Nurse leaders continued to examine nursing and began to look
not just at what nurses were doing but why, how and when.
An early example of such an approach was stimulated by Dr.
Ruth P. Kuehn, dean of the School of Nursing at the University
of Pittsburgh with consultant Dr. Lillian M. Gilbreth as a
member of the advisory committee. Dean Kuehn had begun by
recognizing the need for improving the nursing procedure
manuals current at that time. She soon recognized that not
only did the writing need attention; even more important, the
way nursing procedures were performed needed analysis and
improvement. The initial study was expanded to a three-year
project and became known as "The Hospital Scientific Management Project" (Ganong, 1953).

The focus of study soon shifted from the nurse to nursing and
then to the recipient of nursing—the patient. From these
efforts emerged new concepts about nursing and nursing practice. The components of the nursing process were being

identified. Yura and Walsh (1978b) credit a faculty group at
The Catholic University of America in 1967 with describing the
four steps of the nursing process. A nursing literature review of that period shows emphasis on the concepts and ideas
of what became identified as the nursing process. The nursing
process offers us today a unifying framework for the practice
of nursing.

Components of Nursing

Before we proceed further with our study of the nursing process, it is essential to examine our views about nursing. As
we do this, please realize that nursing is a synergism. None
of the component aspects we examine are "nursing". It is
only when all of the aspects are uniquely orchestrated that
nursing exists. That is why it seems at times so difficult to
examine, describe and define nursing. Recognizing such inherent limitations, we will examine some of these component
aspects.

EXERCISE #1

List all the words you can think of which for you
describe nursing. Compare and contrast your description of nursing with that of several nurse
leaders whose descriptions follow. Which items
are consistently found on the lists?

Florence Nightingale's chapter titles in her Notes on Nursing
provide a clue to the items she considered the essence of
nursing. They are:

Ventilation & warming

Health of houses

Petty management

Noise

Variety

Taking food

What food?

Bed and bedding

Light

Cleanliness of rooms and walls

Personal cleanliness

Chattering hopes and advices

Observations of the sick

6

More recently Virginia Henderson in <u>The Nature of Nursing</u>
noted that "the nurse is the authority on basic nursing care.
By basic I mean helping the patient with the following activities or providing conditions under which he can perform
them unaided:

> Breathe normally
>
> Eat and drink adequately
>
> Eliminate body wastes
>
> Move and maintain desirable postures
>
> Sleep and rest
>
> Select suitable clothes—dress and undress
>
> Maintain body temperature within normal
> range by adjusting clothing and modifying
> the environment
>
> Keep the body clean and well groomed and
> protect the integument
>
> Avoid dangers in the environment and avoid
> injuring others
>
> Communicate with others in expressing emo-
> tions, needs, fears or opinions
>
> Worship according to one's faith
>
> Work in such a way that there is a sense
> of accomplishment
>
> Play or participate in various forms of
> recreation.
>
> Learn, discover, or satisfy the curiosity
> that leads to normal development and health
> and use the available health facilities."

(Henderson, 1966, p. 16)

Fay Abdellah et al (1960) list 21 nursing problems:

> To maintain good hygiene & physical comfort
>
> To promote optimal activity, exercise, rest
> and sleep
>
> To promote safety through prevention of
> accident, injury, or other trauma and through
> the prevention of the spread of infection
>
> To maintain good body mechanics and prevent
> and correct deformities

To facilitate the maintenance of a supply
of oxygen to all body cells

To facilitate the maintenance of nutrition
of all body cells

To facilitate the maintenance of elimination

To facilitate the maintenance of fluid and
electrolyte balance

To recognize the physiological responses of
the body to disease conditions—pathological,
physiological, and compensatory

To facilitate the maintenance of sensory
function

To facilitate the maintenance of regulatory
mechanisms and functions

To identify and accept positive and negative
expressions, feelings, and reactions

To identify and accept the interrelatedness
of emotions and organic illness

To facilitate the maintenance of effective
verbal and nonverbal communication

To promote the development of productive
interpersonal relationships

To facilitate progress toward achievement of
personal spiritual goals

To create and/or maintain a therapeutic
environment

To facilitate awareness of self as an individual with varying physical, emotional, and
developmental needs

To accept the optimum possible goals in the
light of limitations, physical and emotional

To use community resources as an aid in
resolving problems arising from illness

To understand the role of social problems as
influencing factors in the cause of illness

Josephine Paterson, a nursologist (the author's term), presents us with a different kind of list of nursing descriptors (1978, p. 65).

Acceptance	Give-and-take
Authenticity	Laughing-crying
Awareness	Loneliness
Becoming	Openness
Caring	Patience
Change	Readiness
Choice	Response
Commitment	Responsibility
Confirmation	Self-recognition
Confrontation	Sustaining
Dedication	Touching
Dying and death	Trust
Food—its meaning	Understanding
Freedom	Waiting
Frustration	

In these descriptions of nursing you will note that, except for Paterson, they focus primarily on the content of nursing, i.e., the physiological and psychological factors of nursing care. There are other important aspects of the nursing concept, however. One of these is nursing responsibility. To whom and for what are we accountable and responsible in nursing? A profession exists solely in response to a need of society. Nursing exists to fulfill healthcare needs of society's client/patient. The client/patient is nursing's reason for being and must be viewed as the nucleus of nursing.

Nursing's responsibilities can be classified within three areas - care, cure and coordination. Curing appears to be a dominant force in health care. The curative process seeks restoration of health as the ultimate goal. Many nursing activities involve curative measures. Administering medications and treatments are primarily for the purpose of prevention of illness or further sequelae, and for the maintenance or restoration of health. Within the curative domain, nursing assumes both dependent and independent roles. It is the physician's responsibility to provide the orders specifying the medications and treatments to be administered. Nursing actions include carrying out of the orders. Some independence in judgment is required regarding the need for, and the observed results of, such treatment. But the responsibility of the nurse within the curative domain is secondary to that of the physician.

Caring means to be interested and concerned. It involves valuing persons—their human dignity and worth. It requires involvement and a commitment to helping. Note that it is such a part of nursing that we use it frequently to describe nursing—we call it nursing care. Caring permeates all of nursing, and for caring we have primary and independent responsibility. Examine some of the caring activities in providing comfort to the patient and you will realize that we have total independence to select and carry out those measures we determine to be most appropriate for the patient. To reposition, offer a backrub and/or talk with the patient is an exclusive matter of nursing judgment and patient need. The responsibility for nursing <u>care</u> is totally within the domain of nursing.

Our third area of responsibility is that of coordination—coordination of the many activities and services provided the patient in behalf of health care delivery. Scheduling, referring, and talking with any and all of the many health team members is all part of this collaborative function. We might consider this an area of shared responsibility but one that is required of us nonetheless. It has become recognized that the nurse, more than any other member of the health care team, views the person in his/her human wholeness. The focus of each of the other health disciplines is more specific. And so it is appropriate for nursing, as the discipline with this broad perspective, to assume responsibility for the coordination of healthcare. (See also "The head nurse as hospital-integrator," Ganong and Ganong, 1977).

<u>EXERCISE #2</u>
    Refer again to the list of words you made which
    for you described nursing. (See Exercise #1)
    Try to classify each item according to the area
    of responsibility—care, cure, coordination.

In our examination of the components of nursing we have thus far looked at the areas of nursing responsibility, function, and content. Next it seems appropriate to consider methods by which nursing care is provided. Such terms as functional nursing, team nursing, and primary nursing may come to mind. All are recognized,systematic ways by which to organize nursing services for delivery of care. Inherent within each, however, is a basic philosophy and view about just what nursing is.

Ganong and Ganong (1975b, p. 12) note that the performance of nurses is influenced inevitably by how they view themselves and their roles. These perceptions of self and role are the result of many factors. One of these factors is the way in which nurses are educated and oriented. Edith P. Lewis, editor of <u>Nursing Outlook</u>, provides this succinct summary.

> *To the student we say, "This is your*
> *patient;" to the staff nurse, "This is*
> *your job." Small wonder that in the*
> *transition from the one to the other*
> *the nurse ends up by devaluing the pa-*
> *tient, herself, and the job.*

In the diagram "Two Views of Nursing" (Figure 2), two contrasting concepts of the nursing role are presented. Concept A is the Nursing Workload Concept in which the patients are seen as generating a daily volume of routine work to be done through the performance of necessary tasks and procedures. The question sometimes heard on the nursing unit, "Do you have your patients done yet?" symbolizes Concept A. Concept B is the Patient Care Management Concept. Here the client is seen as a person with identified needs and problems for which he seeks help. He (insofar as he is able) participates with his family (or significant others), his doctor, and his nurse to develop the goal(s) for his care together with the objectives that must be met to achieve the goal. The relevant day-to-day question now is "How well is the client meeting his objectives?" (Ganong & Ganong, 1975b).

Idealistic? Yes! Possible? Yes! How? By use of the nursing process a patient care orientation and approach can be achieved. The process begins when the patient enters the healthcare system for care. Initial assessment directs attention to the individual and his specific needs. Development and implementation of a plan of care continues focus on the primary needs of the patient. Evaluation of results helps to assure continued focus on individual needs and problems. The "Components of Nursing" model (Figure 3) helps one visualize the elements of nursing.

Concept A: <u>NURSING WORKLOAD CONCEPT</u>

("Do you have your patients done yet?")

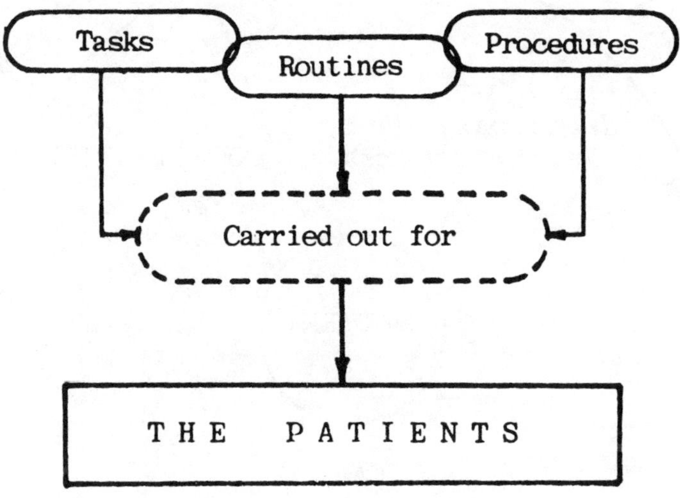

Concept B: <u>PATIENT CARE MANAGEMENT CONCEPT</u>

("How well is the client meeting his objectives?")

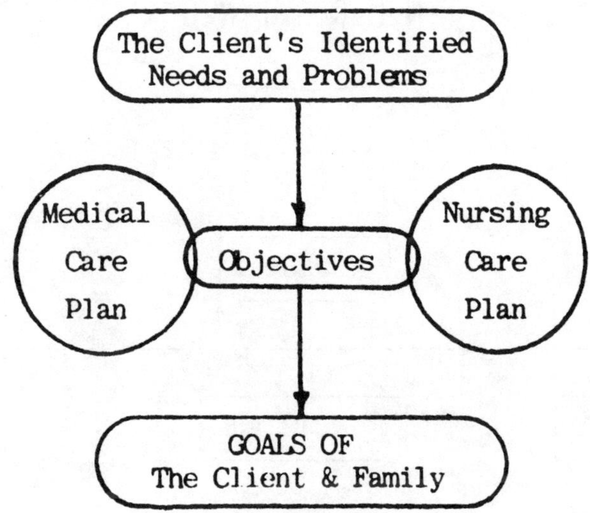

FIGURE 2

Source: Ganong, J., & Ganong, W. L. <u>HELP with the problem-oriented nursing system</u>. Chapel Hill, NC: W. L. Ganong Company, 1975, p. 12. Used with permission.

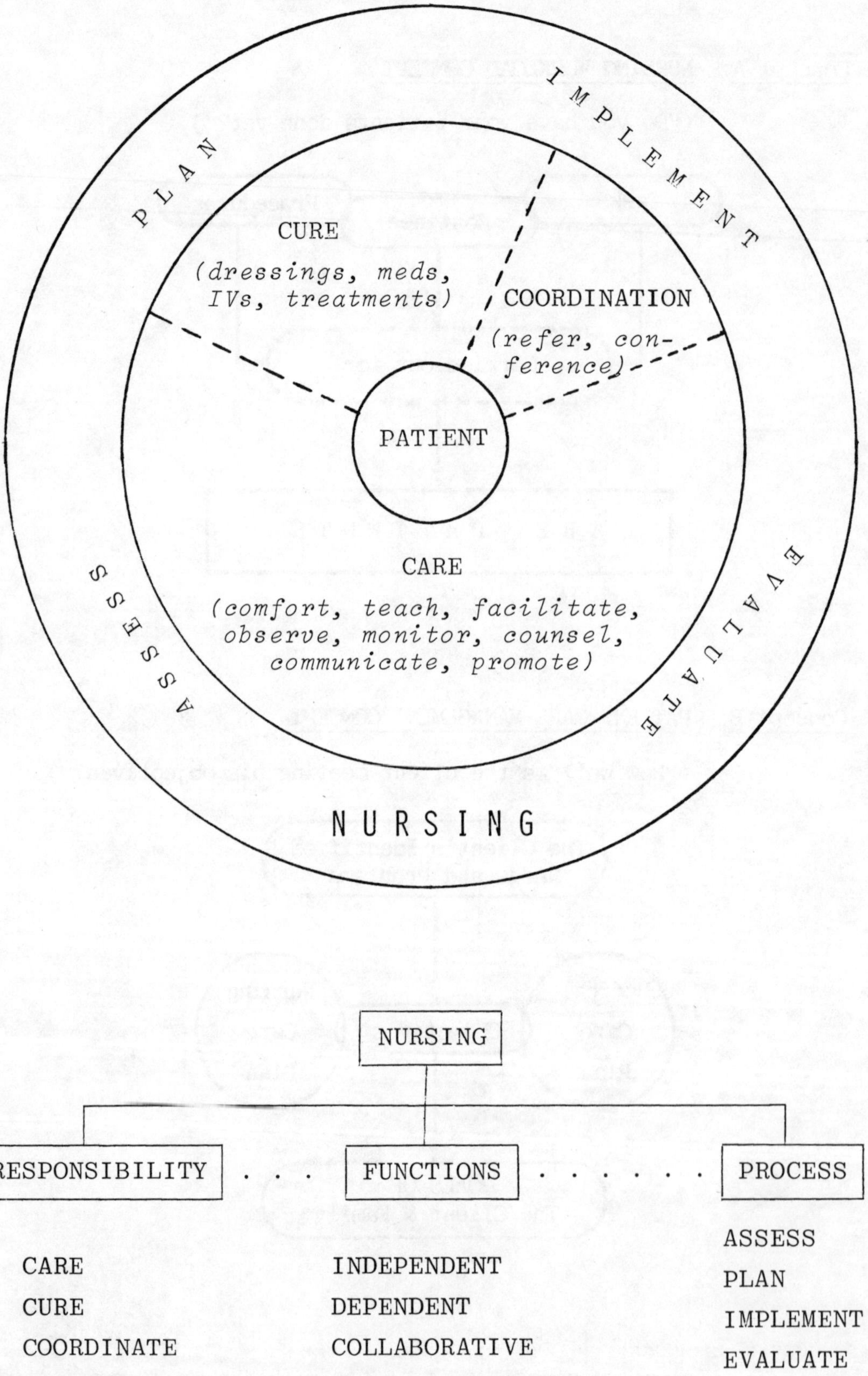

PLAN
IMPLEMENT
CURE
(dressings, meds, IVs, treatments)
COORDINATION
(refer, conference)
PATIENT
CARE
(comfort, teach, facilitate, observe, monitor, counsel, communicate, promote)
ASSESS
EVALUATE
NURSING
NURSING
RESPONSIBILITY
FUNCTIONS
PROCESS
CARE
CURE
COORDINATE
INDEPENDENT
DEPENDENT
COLLABORATIVE
ASSESS
PLAN
IMPLEMENT
EVALUATE

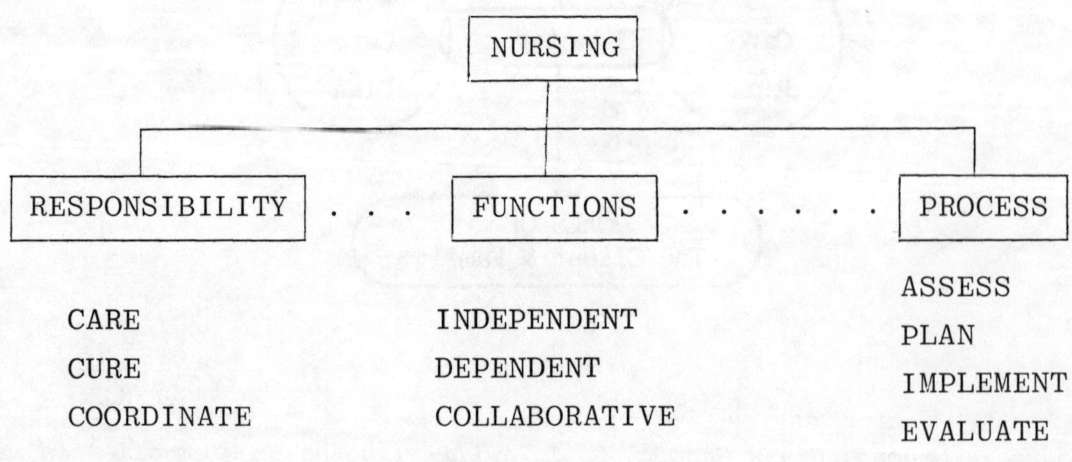

COMPONENTS OF NURSING

Figure 3

Benefits of the Nursing Process

1. Meet individual patient needs

2. Give more complete care

3. Be more systematic in giving care

4. Make better use of scientific principles

5. Be accountable for care

6. Set appropriate priorities for care

7. Usable in any setting with any type of patient/client

EXERCISE #3

Review each of the seven benefits of the nursing process. Give an example of how the use of the nursing process will achieve each of the benefits.

Nursing Practice

Having examined some of the major components of nursing, let us now look at some available guides that can assist us in nursing practice. See the following six pages.

The professional organization (American Nurses Association) first developed a model Nurse Practice Act in 1955. The latest revision (1976) is as follows:

> *The practice of nursing as performed by a registered nurse is a process in which substantial specialized knowledge derived from the biological, physical and behavioral sciences is applied to the care, treatment, counsel and health teaching of persons who are experiencing changes in the normal health processes, or who require assistance in the maintenance of health or the management of illness, injury, or infirmity or in the achievement of a dignified death, and such additional acts as are recognized by the nursing profession as proper to be performed by a registered nurse.*

In-depth study of these documents reveals that the nursing process is inherent in each. The nursing profession as well as regulatory bodies such as the Joint Commission on Accreditation of Hospitals subscribe to the nursing process as the means by which nursing is to be practiced.

The practice of nursing today requires an individual who possesses unique capabilities. She or he must be intelligent, skillful in both technical and interpersonal matters, in command of change, and committed to nursing.

PREAMBLE: The Code for Nurses is based on belief about
                    the nature of individuals, nursing, health,
                    and society. Recipients and providers of
                    nursing services are viewed as individuals
                    and groups who possess basic rights and re-
                    sponsibilities, and whose values and circum-
                    stances command respect at all times. Nurs-
                    ing encompasses the promotion and restoration
                    of health, the prevention of illness, and the
                    alleviation of suffering. The statements of
                    the Code and their interpretation provide
                    guidance for conduct and relationships in
                    carrying out nursing responsibilities consis-
                    tent with the ethical obligations of the pro-
                    fession and quality in nursing care.

CODE FOR NURSES: 1. The nurse provides services with respect for
                       human dignity and the uniqueness of the client
                       unrestricted by considerations of social or
                       economic status, personal attributes, or the
                       nature of health problems.
                   2. The nurse safeguards the client's right to pri-
                       vacy by judiciously protecting information of
                       a confidential nature.
                   3. The nurse acts to safeguard the client and the
                       public when healthcare and safety are affected
                       by the incompetent, unethical, or illegal prac-
                       tice of any person.
                   4. The nurse assumes responsibility and accounta-
                       bility for individual nursing judgments and
                       actions.
                   5. The nurse maintains competence in nursing.
                   6. The nurse exercises informed judgment and uses
                       individual competence and qualifications as
                       criteria in seeking consultation, accepting re-
                       sponsibilities, and delegating nursing activities
                       to others.
                   7. The nurse participates in activities that contri-
                       bute to the ongoing development of the pro-
                       fession's body of knowledge.
                   8. The nurse participates in the profession's ef-
                       forts to implement and improve standards of
                       nursing.
                   9. The nurse participates in the profession's ef-
                       forts to establish and maintain conditions of
                       employment conducive to high quality nursing
                       care.
                  10. The nurse participates in the profession's ef-
                       fort to protect the public from misinformation
                       and misrepresentation and to maintain the integ-
                       rity of nursing.
                  11. The nurse collaborates with members of the
                       health professions and other citizens in
                       promoting community and national efforts to
                       meet the health needs of the public.

Source: *Code for nurses with interpretative statements,* *American Nurses*
Association, Kansas City, Mo. 1979. Used with permission of ANA.

Preamble

The Council on Practice recognizes its responsibility for articulating the role of nursing practice within the health care delivery system. In order for the Council to speak effectively about nursing practice, it is apparent that a framework explaining practice and its contributions to the health care of citizens is desirable and necessary.

Traditionally, nursing has been discussed in terms of behaviors of practitioners rather than the process involved in practice. Since the Council's formation, it has examined nursing practice and the contributions of practitioners to the total health care delivery system. Accordingly, the Council on Practice has developed a statement emphasizing the the client's rights regarding nursing care.

Statement

Nursing practice has a distinct responsibility for the promotion of, restoration to, and maintenance of a specified state of health of its clients that include individuals, families, groups, and communities. Nursing practice encompasses physiological, psychosocial, cultural, and environmental aspects and relates them to the total unity of the client. Because of its focus on health as well as on deviations from health, nursing practice is appropriate in all client settings. Further, the amount of nursing practice is determined by the client's state of integrity and ability to promote, restore, and maintain health.

Nursing practice shares with other health professions responsibility for health needs of society. This shared responsibility mandates continuing endeavors to define health; to determine the human and material resources necessary to meet health needs; and to contribute to the surveillance and improvement of the environment so that promotion, restoration, and maintenance of health take place.

Nursing practice is affected by delegated responsibility for activities commonly seen as those within the purview of other health professions. These activities constitute horizontal delegation among health professions with mutual accountability for completion of the specified activities. Acceptance by nursing of delegated responsibility requires specification of a nursing goal.

The health care delivery system which is accessible, available, and feasible, is composed of several health professions working for the health of all persons.

Nursing practice is integrated within the health care delivery system and is responsible for nursing practice decisions and their consequences. Hence, nursing practice is accountable to the client.

The role of nursing practice is based upon the expectation that this practice will contribute to the client's unity. The nursing practice is based upon scientific knowledge and established criteria for competence. The client has the right to expect that the nursing practice is made a matter of record and is goal-directed, based upon specified client requirements. The goal-directed actions, in practice, are reflective of the following process:

Assessment   Assessment includes the systematic collection of data under the categories of physiological, psychosocial, cultural, and environmental observable aspects of the client.

The data are collected from individuals, families, groups, and communities as well as from material resources. The data are analyzed, compared with normative values, and organized into a logical pattern. Facts, opinions, and values are distinguished; relationships and conclusions are stated and documented.

Planning   Planning includes specification of logical progression of short to long-term goals; description of alternative nursing actions and the consequences to each of the alternatives; determination of priorities; and the statement of the rationale for selected nursing actions. Planning of nursing practice goals is done with the client or with those persons responsible for the client. Other health professions serve as resources, directly or indirectly, in the planning.

Implementation   The goal-directed nursing plan is implemented in the most effective and efficient way possible. The nursing actions include, but are not limited to, such means as giving and/or providing care, communicating, teaching, leading, and interacting. Modification of these actions takes into account those factors that alter the planned implementation; and incorporates the processes of assessment, planning, and evaluation for justification of specified modifications. Nursing actions are documented.

Evaluation   Evaluation is an ongoing process which reflects stated purpose(s), standards of nursing practice, and the use of appropriate methodology. Effectiveness of nursing practice is systematically evaluated.

THE NURSING PROCESS
and the
PRESENT LEGAL AND JUDICIAL PATTERNS OF IDENTIFYING
PROFESSIONAL NURSING AREAS OF CONTROL,
FUNCTION AND RESPONSIBILITY

1. Supervision of the patient including total management of his/her nursing care by use of the <u>assessment</u> or interview to identify patient problems and <u>plan</u> for their alleviation or their elimination.

2. Supervision and teaching of others participating in his/her care by providing a <u>plan</u> of nursing care with specific directives to guide the nursing team.

3. Application and execution of nursing procedures and techniques to <u>implement</u> the nursing action necessary.

4. Promotion and maintenance of physical and emotional health as well as prevention of illness of patient and/or family by direction and <u>teaching</u>.

5. Observation of symptoms and reactions, both physical and mental, and <u>interpreting</u> or making decisions about the patient's response to their illness or treatment.

6. Accurate recording and reporting of facts, including <u>evaluation</u> of total care that the patient received as well as reflections in the patient's progress notes as to effectiveness or ineffectiveness of nursing care planned.

7. Application and execution of licensed physician or dentists' prescribed orders concerning treatments and medications, or diagnostic evaluation.

Both the areas of professional nursing are based on the fact that the professional nurse <u>must</u> understand cause and effect at all times whether functioning in the dependent or independent areas.

Adapted from: Lesnik and Anderson, <u>Nursing Practice and the Law</u>, p. 259-282, 1955.
1962 Report of ANA's Committee on Legislation, JCAH, Standards, 1970.

Source: Vasey, E., & Reilly, M. <u>Quality assurance: Peer review for nursing</u>. Western Penn. RMP, Nursing Division, Pittsburgh, PA 1975. Used with permission.

AMERICAN NURSES' ASSOCIATION
STANDARDS OF NURSING PRACTICE

STANDARD I

The collection of data about the health status of the client/
patient is systematic and continuous. The data are accessible, communicated, and recorded.

STANDARD II

Nursing diagnoses are derived from health status data.

STANDARD III

The plan of nursing care includes goals derived from the
nursing diagnoses.

STANDARD IV

The plan of nursing care includes priorities and the prescribed nursing approaches or measures to achieve the goals
derived from the nursing diagnoses.

STANDARD V

Nursing actions provide for client/patient participation in
health promotion, maintenance and restoration.

STANDARD VI

Nursing actions assist the client/patient to maximize his
health capabilities.

STANDARD VII

The client's/patient's progress or lack of progress toward
goal achievement is determined by the client/patient and the
nurse.

STANDARD VIII

The client's/patient's progress or lack of progress toward
goal achievement directs reassessment, reordering of priorities, new goal setting and revision of the plan of nursing
care.

JCAH NURSING SERVICE STANDARDS   (1980)

STANDARD I

The nursing department/service shall be directed by a quali-
fied nurse administrator and shall be appropriately integrated
with the medical staff and with other hospital staffs that
provide and contribute to patient care.

STANDARD II

The nursing department/service shall be organized to meet the
nursing care needs of patients and to maintain established
standards of nursing practice.

STANDARD III

Nursing department/service assignments in the provision of
nursing care shall be commensurate with the qualifications of
nursing personnel and shall meet the nursing care needs of
patients.

STANDARD IV

Individualized, goal-directed nursing care shall be provided
to patients through the use of the nursing process.

STANDARD V

Nursing department/service personnel shall be prepared through
appropriate education and training programs for their responsibilities in the provision of nursing care.

STANDARD VI

Written policies and procedures that reflect optimal standards
of nursing practice shall guide the provision of nursing care.

STANDARD VII

The nursing department/service shall provide mechanisms for
the regular review and evaluation of the quality and appropriateness of nursing department/service practice and functions. Such mechanisms shall be designed to attain optimal
achievable standards of nursing care.

NURSING PROCESS

RESPONSE SHEET #2

Read each statement. Circle A (Agree), D (Disagree), or
? (Not sure) to indicate your response. Be prepared to explain your decisions. There are not necessarily any right
or wrong answers.

A   D   ?   1. It is possible to perform each step of the
                    nursing process when caring for a patient
                    regardless of his specific nursing needs or
                    the setting in which care is delivered.

A   D   ?   2. Nursing process is based on the scientific
                    principles of problem-solving.

A   D   ?   3. Nursing process helps the nurse better meet
                    the individual needs of patients.

A   D   ?   4. Nursing has both dependent and independent
                    areas of practice.

A   D   ?   5. Nursing has three areas of responsibility—
                    care, cure and coordination.

A   D   ?   6. Nursing process is used continuously from
                    the time of admission to discharge of the
                    patient.

A   D   ?   7. The steps of nursing process are assessment,
                    planning, implementation, and evaluation.

A   D   ?   8. Nurses frequently view nursing as a series
                    of tasks and procedures to be completed
                    rather than a process of care.

A   D   ?   9. "What is Nursing?" can best be answered by
                    listing what nurses do.

A   D   ?   10. Nursing process directs nursing practice.

<u>HELP</u> WITH ASSESSMENT

*The collection of data about the health status of the client/patient is sys-
tematic and continuous: the data are accessible, communicated and recorded.*

ANA Standards of Practice, 1973

Introduction

Assessment is a relatively new nursing term for many nurses, but one being used with increasing frequency. It does not have a universally accepted definition. In the context of this study manual, it refers to
the initial step of the nursing process.

> Assessment is defined as the systematic gathering of in-
> formation about a patient's health and illness, then
> analyzing the information using nursing knowledge and
> judgment to determine individual patient problems and
> needs for nursing care. Note in this definition that
> two major activities are described within assessment,
> information gathering and analyzing. Both require
> unique skills and ability on the part of the nurse.

The nursing process begins with assessing. The remaining three phases—
planning, implementing, and evaluating—are totally dependent upon the
quality and completeness of the initial assessment and ongoing reassessment. Thus it is essential not only that assessment be done but that
the results be presented in a systematic, accessible, timely and useful
fashion.

Data Collection: First Step

The gathering of health information about the patient/client sometimes
begins even before the first interaction between nurse and patient, for
there are various sources from which the information can be collected.
This data collection activity is referred to by a variety of terms such
as "taking a nursing history", "doing a patient assessment", or just
"assessing". Common sources for patient assessment information include:
the patient; physicians, nurses and other healthcare workers; family
and friends; records and reports.

To assure a complete assessment, nurses gather data from as many sources
as possible. Success in conducting the assessment is greatly dependent
upon the nurse's communication skills. Highly important among these
are observing, interviewing, and listening. A significant amount of
information can be gathered through observation. Some "Tips on Observation" are included herewith.

A Tip: *Useful information; helpful hints.*

To Observe is: *To watch attentively; to perceive; to take notice; to pay attention.*

Observing a patient means to pay attention through the use of your senses—sight, hearing, smell, touch. Observing also means being alert to the *feeling tones* you get from a person.

A. The Use of Your Senses

1. Look for signs and symptoms of potential problems such as a rash, a tremor, bleeding, a bruise, broken skin, swelling, crying.

2. Watch facial expressions to pick up clues about such things as fatigue, fear, doubt, anxiety, satisfaction, anger, hostility, pain, confidence.

3. Watch body posture and position for clues about the same things mentioned in 2.

4. Read in the bibliography at the end of this manual for further help.

5. Listen for breath sounds, the timbre of a person's voice, the emphasis placed on words, for unspoken questions and needs.

6. Smell for odors that emanate from the patient's body— his breath, drainage from a wound or body orifice.

B. General Guidelines

1. Remember that it is easy to *see* without *observing*, so pay attention to detail.

2. Observe for signs and symptoms based upon pre-determined criteria.

3. Observe by looking at the patient holistically.

4. Take time to be receptive to what your senses tell you; observe receptively.

5. As you observe the patient, remember that *what* is observed depends on you. What you *see* may be what you *expect to see.*

6. People's behavior stems from their interpretation of what they think they perceive.

7. It helps to *practice observing silently* to allow all of your receptive senses to function without the interference of your own voice.

8. Observing includes reading. You can observe for information. Refer to the bibliography for further help.

9. Record observations made.

Source: *Ganong, J. and Ganong, W. Tips on observing.* HELP with a problem-oriented nursing system. *W.L. Ganong Co., Chapel Hill, NC, 1975. p. 63-64.*

The following outline illustrates some observations to be made using your senses of seeing, hearing, touching, and smelling.

Observations Using Your Senses

Observations made by seeing—

Client/patient:	general appearance, behavior, visible physical factors, clothing, habits, attachments and prostheses
Surrounding environment:	personal possessions, home environment, family and significant others

Observations made by hearing—

Client/patient:	voice and speech; breathing; heart, lung, and abdominal sounds
Surrounding environment:	noises (both usual and unusual)

Observations made by touching—

Client/patient:	head (lumps, hair texture), skin (temperature, pulsations), chest (masses), abdomen (muscle tension)
Surrounding environment:	dressings, bedding, equipment

Observations made by smelling—

Client/patient:	perspiration, discharges from body orifices and wounds, breath odor, use of chemicals
Surrounding environment:	food odors, "hospital" and other odors of the surroundings.

In addition to observing, much assessment information will be collected by interview. An interview involves much more than talking. It is purposeful and goal-directed. Practice the following "Tips on Interviewing" to enhance your interviewing skills.

A Tip: *Useful information; helpful hints.*

An interview is *a face-to-face meeting for conversation to obtain information.*

> Interviewing is a communications process. Communication
> is the creation of understanding. A variety of skills
> are involved. How these skills are used depends upon
> the purpose, perception, and ability of the interviewer.

A. <u>General Guidelines</u>

1. The climate you set influences the interview.

    a. Show a sincere interest in what the patient is saying;
        listen attentively.

    b. Trust is established by proximity, responsiveness,
        openness, attention, privacy, confidentiality, honesty.

    c. Determine the patient's habits, feelings, and know-
        ledge as effectively and efficiently and as pleasantly
        as possible.

    d. An attitude of warm acceptance and understanding coupled
        with objectivity will enhance the results of an inter-
        view.

    e. Introduce yourself by name and title, and tell the
        patient the reason for the interview.

    f. Be seated comfortably during the interview.

2. Always use the data base form to record accurately the in-
    formation as the patient gives it to you. Do not rely on
    your memory.

3. Remember that the needs and goals of both patient and
    nurse determine the purpose and outcome of an interview.

4. Do not ask questions of the patient that are already
    answered elsewhere--unless it is necessary to check for
    accuracy.

5. It is the responsibility of the interviewer to keep the
    interview on the track.

6. Observe the patient for fatigue; pace the interview
    accordingly.

7. Practice interviewing. This will refine your use of the
    technique and help you identify and correct weak spots
    in your own skills. The more interviews you do, the more
    adept you can become.

Tips on Interviewing (Cont.)

B.   Use of Questions

    1.   Use direct questions to get specific information.
         "What is your age?" "When were you born?"
    2.   Use exploratory questions to encourage further comments and expression of feelings.
         "How do you feel about that?" "Would you tell me more about that?"
    3.   Use open-ended questions to allow person to comment about whatever is on his mind.
         "What would you like to talk about?" "What can I do to make you more comfortable?"

C.   Listening

    1.   Listen for facts and for meanings.

    2.   Concentrate on the patient and what he is saying.

    3.   Don't be afraid of silence. Wait long enough for the patient to respond in his own way.

    4.   Listen; then write. Take time for eye contact.

    5.   Listen responsively and thoughtfully.

    6.   Remember: *meanings are in people, not in words.*

D.   Other Communication Skills

    Use the sum total of all your verbal and non-verbal communication skills during an interview. People use the movements of their head, arms, eyes and torso to punctuate their speech—and to communicate additional meanings.

Source: Ganong J. and Ganong, W. "Tips on Interviewing". HELP with a Problem-Oriented Nursing System. W.L. Ganong Co., Chapel Hill, NC, 1975, p. 61-62.

Listening

The skill of listening is often poorly used by nurses. As the Ganongs (1976) state, "Listening is difficult; listening takes time; listening is hard work; listening is tiring. Listening skill is essential, however, and it can be developed." Good listening is a key to success in interviewing. Creative listening is a technique nurses should know and use. Assess your listening skills using the following pages.

DETERMINE WHAT IS OF VALUE TO YOU PERSONALLY

Select the important from the unimportant.
Sift out the wheat from the chaff.

ALWAYS LISTEN FOR CENTRAL IDEAS

Train yourself to seek the main idea—key points.

IDENTIFY AND DECREASE THE NUMBER OF YOUR PSYCHOLOGICAL OR EMOTIONAL DEAF SPOTS.

Isolate any important prejudices you may have which
might serve to distort your thinking.

EXPLOIT THE ADVANTAGE OF THOUGHT SPEED OVER SPEECH SPEED BY:

1. Anticipation - Look ahead.
2. Discrimination - Evaluate and sift.
3. Recapitulation - Summarize and review.
4. Look for hidden meanings.

It is possible for any of us to learn more by listening than
many ever learn by reading or talking.

LISTEN ACTIVELY - NOT PASSIVELY

To be a good listener one must develop his concentration—
perhaps the most important aid to good listening.

IT TAKES ENERGY TO LISTEN

Being a good listener pays off in better understanding,
closer friendships, increased efficiency—perhaps even
a salary increase.

The art of listening remains one of the "most overlooked tools
of management." It is the least efficient of our communication
skills.

*Source: Ganong, J., & Ganong, W. HELP with the results-oriented performance
evaluation program. Chapel Hill, NC: W. L. Ganong Co. 1974, p. 81.*

	Yes	No

1. As patients talk to you, do you find it difficult
    to keep your mind on the subject at hand, to keep
    from taking mental excursions away from the line of
    thought that is being conveyed?

2. Do you listen primarily for facts, rather than
    ideas, when the patient is speaking?

3. Do certain words, phrases or ideas so prejudice you
    against a patient that you cannot listen objective-
    ly to what is being said?

4. When you are puzzled or annoyed by what the
    patient says, do you try to get the question
    straightened out immediately, either in your own
    mind or by interrupting the patient?

5. If you feel it would take too much time and effort
    to understand something, do you go out of your way
    to avoid hearing about it?

6. Do you deliberately turn your thoughts to other
    subjects when you believe a patient will have
    nothing particularly interesting to say?

7. Can you tell by the patient's appearance and de-
    livery that he/she won't have anything worthwhile
    to say?

8. When a patient is talking to you, do you try to
    make him/her think you are paying attention when
    you are not?

9. When you are listening to a patient, are you
    easily distracted by outside sights and sounds?

10. If you really want to remember what the patient
    is saying, do you try to write down most of what
    is being said?

THE ASSESSMENT MAN

To observe accurately is one thing, to organize data rapidly and logically is another. To do both students need a compact tool and on-the-spot experience in using it at the bedside.

HELEN WOLFF ● ROBERTA ERICKSON

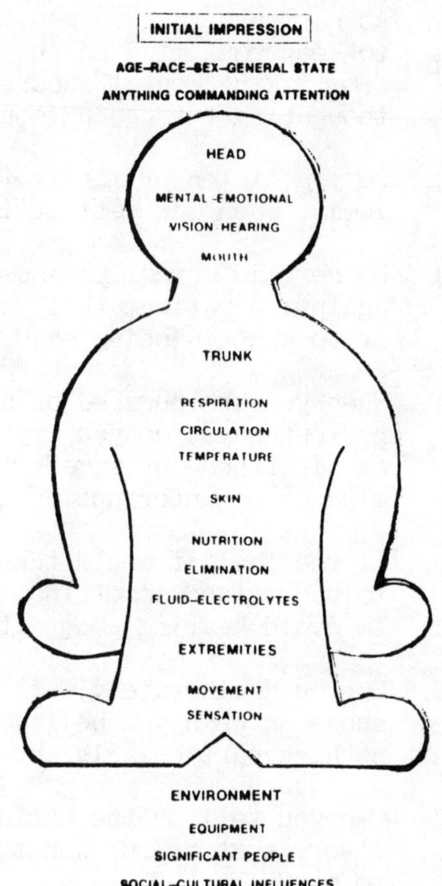

But if you cannot get the habit of observation one way or another you had better give up the being a nurse, for it is not your calling, however kind and anxious you may be.

Florence Nightingale
Notes on nursing

This is an on-the-spot assessment experience designed to provide immediate reinforcement of your bedside observations and nursing care planning ability.

You will have 10 minutes to assess a selected patient. You may use any tools (stethoscope, etc.), senses, physical examination techniques, communication skills, or other abilities that you have. Any information available in the patient's room is acceptable for use. You may not look at the chart or Kardex or discuss observations and care with others.

At the end of the assessment period, meet immediately with your instructor. List all observations you made, state the patient's nursing care problems and your goals for care (identify priorities), describe specific nursing actions to accomplish each goal (assume you have any needed medical orders), summarize the reasoning behind the actions, and outline any additional information you would require to provide total nursing care for the patient.

Figure 4

<u>Improving Physical Assessment Skills</u>

Many nurses are expanding their skills in physical assessment.
Using the methods of inspection, palpation, percussion, and
auscultation and becoming more adept in the use of equipment
such as the stethoscope and otoscope, they are able to gather
more indepth physiological data with which to plan nursing
care. Several kinds of data are needed for a complete assessment, and accurate physiological data is essential. Two
common approaches to the collection of physiological data are
by a review of body systems or by a head-to-toe review. Wolff
and Erickson (1977) provide a useful tool for conducting head-
to-toe assessment; they call it "The Assessment Man". (See Figure 4).

In addition to physiological data, it is also important to
gather psychological information. Such things as the patient's
mental and emotional status, orientation, mood, and body
image should be assessed. Attitudes, behaviors—especially
non-verbal cues and feelings—should be noted. Social factors
such as life-style, home environment, family relationships
and support, employment and/or occupation, past experiences
with illness and/or health care, likes and dislikes, and
habits provide unique and essential information about the
patient. The cultural influences of language, customs, beliefs, values, religion, and diet are also important areas to
be assessed in order to recognize and provide for needs specific to the patient.

Major types of information needed, therefore, in order to
have a complete assessment are:

- Physiological data
- Psychological data
- Social data
- Cultural data

The specific information gathered within each category will
vary depending upon the patient's reasons for seeking health
care, the setting, and the nature of nursing care being
provided. For example, relevant assessment data about an em-
ployee seeking the services of an occupational health nurse
for an industrial accident will be considerably different
from the type of appropriate information needed about a home-
bound chronically ill individual or a patient admitted to
the hospital for major abdominal surgery. Appropriate data
within each of the four types, however, will be needed and
should be identified.

32

The gathering of assessment data should be done in a complete
and efficient manner. This is best accomplished through the
use of a guide that systematically orders the information.
Most agencies have developed a specific tool or format to be
used for the initial assessment. Length is quite varied.
There is no one best type of assessment form but there are
some important considerations in its design.

<u>Guidelines for Developing Assessment Tools</u>

1. Determine the purpose for which the assessment tool is
    to be used

    Consider: What is the setting? (hospital, nursing home,
                                      ambulatory clinic, home
                                      health, etc.)

                 What type of patient? (adult, child, medical,
                                        surgical, etc.)

                 When is assessment done? (initial admission;
                                           reassessments)

2. Select the content

    Consider: Is data to be comprehensive? (body systems,
                                               head-to-toe, etc.)

                 Is data to be specific? (focus on particular
                                          clinical diagnosis,
                                          nursing problem, patient
                                          population, etc.)

3. Design the format

    Consider: Style (Outline, completion statement, check-
                        lists, ratings)

                 Length (Number of pages)

                 Arrangement and order of content items

4. Pilot test a draft of the assessment tool

    Consider: Where to pilot test

                 Who to pilot test

                 When to pilot test

                 How long to pilot test

                 Method for gathering responses, suggestions,
                 recommendations

                 How to evaluate the pilot test

5. Make indicated changes in the tool based upon findings
    of the pilot test

    Consider: Users' responses, suggestions, recommendations

                 Pilot test evaluation results

6. Plan for adoption and implementation of the assessment
    tool

    Consider: Staff orientation needs

                 Policies and procedures to be written or revised

                 When to initiate adoption.

For examples of specific assessment tools and formats, refer
to the Ganongs' <u>HELP with a Problem-Oriented Nursing System</u>
(pp. 65-70). Remember that while none of these samples may be
appropriate for your use without revision, they may provide
helpful ideas of style, content and format.

<u>EXERCISE #4:   Unstructured and Structured Assessments</u>
    The purpose of this exercise is to illustrate the bene-
    fits and limitations of both structured and unstructured
    assessments. Select a partner who will be the patient/
    client. You are the nurse. In the next few minutes find
    out all you can about this person's health (allow 5-6
    minutes). Summarize what you learned about the indivi-
    dual's health.

                            then

Keep the same partner and roles. Conduct another health
assessment using the following guide.

1. Observe the person and write down a few key words
    of description.

2. Ask the person: Describe yourself

                     Describe your state of health—
                     illnesses and diseases past and
                     present; family illness and dis-
                     ease; how often off work in past
                     year, for what reasons

                     Describe your eating pattern & diet

                     What exercise do you engage in?

                     What do you do for relaxation?

                     How much rest & sleep do you need? Get?

                     Name something stressful to you.

3. Summarize what you learned about the individual's
    health.

Discuss the following questions:

1. In which type interview did you gather the most
    health information about the individual? Why?

2. What were the advantages you found in an unstructured
    interview? A structured interview?

3. What were the limitations you found in an unstruc-
    tured interview? A structured interview?

EXERCISE #5: Critiquing an Assessment Tool
    Select an assessment tool (preferably one you have
    used) and critique it using the following criteria:

Criteria for an Assessment Tool

1. Its specific purpose (type of tool) is evident.

2. It is systematic; items are in a logical order.

3. Data is presented in a useful, informative manner.

4. It provides for completeness of data.

5. Significant findings can be easily identified.

6. It can be completed with relative ease.

7. It can be done within a reasonable amount of time.

8. It provides for a summary of findings and conclu-
    sions.

9. It is used for developing the plan of care.

10. There are written guidelines explaining its use.

11. It contains a place for the nurse assessor's
    signature.

Analysis of Data: Second Step

The data collection activities of assessment are vitally important. But we must remember this is only one part of the assessment phase of the nursing process. Since the advent of the nursing process, a great amount of focus has been directed on data gathering activities—developing assessment tools, conducting admission interviews (frequently referred to as "doing assessment") and documenting such data. Too frequently the nursing staff believe assessment to be finished when these initial steps are completed. Such is not so. Only when use is made of the information collected is the purpose of assessment realized. In other words, information is not collected for information's sake nor simply to allow us the sense of accomplishment for having completed yet another nursing task.

Information is gathered for the sole purpose of enabling the nurse to be aware of individual patient's specific health needs and problems. Only then can we plan and provide nursing care appropriate to the patient. In order for that to happen, something must be done with the information collected. That "something" is termed analysis—examining the information to interpret and determine its significance.

Analysis requires the skill and expertise of a registered professional nurse. Some nurses have not appreciated the importance and significance of the assessment phase of the nursing process and thus have literally "sold nursing's birthright" by not assuming responsibility and accountability for this important nursing function. Many persons, including the supportive healthcare personnel, can greatly assist the professional nurse in carrying out assessment—particularly with selected data collection activities. But only the professional nurse can and must analytically process all the information gathered to make judgments and decisions for nursing care and its implementation.

Nursing practice standards (of the American Nurses Association, the Joint Commission on Accreditation of Hospitals — JCAH, and the Medicare Conditions of Participation of the Social Security Administration) emphasize assessment functions of registered nurses.

> *Comprehensive care requires complete and*
> *ongoing collection of data about the client/*
> *patient to determine the nursing care needs*
> *of the client/patient.*
>
> > Rationale, Standard I
> > ANA Standards of Nursing
> > Practice, 1973

> *Each patient's nursing needs shall be*
> *assessed by the registered nurse at the*
> *time of admission or within the period*
> *established by nursing department/ser-*
> *vice policy.*
>
> > Interpretation, Standard IV
> > JCAH Nursing Services
> > Standards, 1980

> *The registered nurse makes the initial*
> *evaluation (assessment) visit, regularly*
> *reevaluates the patients nursing needs, . . .*
>
> > Skilled Nursing Service #405.1224
> > Conditions of Participation for
> > Home Health Agencies, 1975

The analysis process is primarily an intellectual activity. There is very little visible behavior during this process. But the end result catapults you into the second phase of the nursing process—planning. In order to analyze efficiently and effectively, the data must be categorized meaningfully. The logical arrangement of content on the assessment guide greatly assists with this task. The nurse, however, categorizes in additional ways. This involves relating bits and pieces of data to compare and contrast them with normal values, using scientific principles to identify factors of signifi-cance, and associating several factors to identify meaningful patterns and trends.

Questions for Analysis

Here are some questions to assist the nurse with the analytical process:

1. What are the significant physiological occurrences?

2. What are the significant psychological occurrences?

3. What clinical signs and symptoms are present?

4. What is happening to the patient socially, culturally, emotionally?

5. What feelings is the patient expressing?

6. What appears to be unusual, atypical, unexpected?

7. How is the patient/family coping.

<u>Nursing Diagnosis</u>

Nursing diagnosis is the term used to describe the outcome of the analytical step of nursing assessment (Block, 1974; Gebbie & Lavin, 1975; Gordon, 1976; Marriner, 1979). The entire October 1979 issue of <u>Advances in Nursing Science</u> was devoted to the topic of nursing diagnosis. Three national conferences on the Classification of Nursing Diagnosis have been held. Work continues on the identification of acceptable diagnostic nomenclature. The diagnostic nomenclature currently accepted is shown in Table 1.

TABLE 1
Areas of Diagnostic Nomenclature Currently Accepted

Anxiety	Nutritional alteration
Bowel elimination, alteration in	Parenting, alterations in
Cardiac output, alteration in	Respiratory dysfunction
Comfort, alterations in	Role disturbance
Consciousness, altered levels of	Self-care activities, alterations in
Coping patterns, maladaptive (individual)	Self-concept, alterations in
Coping, ineffective family	Sensory-perceptual alteration
Digestion, impairment of	Sexuality, alteration in patterns of
Family process, inadequate	Skin integrity, impairment of
Fear	Sleep-rest activity, dysrhythm
Fluid volume, alteration in	Spirituality, matters of
Grieving	Social isolation
Home maintenance management, impaired	Suffocation, potential for
Injury, potential for	Thought processes, impaired
Knowledge, lack of (specify)	Tissue perfusion, chronic abnormal
Manipulation	Trauma, potential for
Mobility, impairment of	Urinary elimination, impairment of
Noncompliance (specify)	Verbal communication, impairment of

Sources: Gebbie, K. M. and Lavin, M.A., eds. *Proceedings of the First National Conference: Classification of Nursing Diagnoses* (St. Louis: The C.V. Mosby Co. 1975).

Gebbie, K. M., ed. *Summary of the Second National Conference on Classification of Nursing Diagnoses* (St. Louis: Clearinghouse for Nursing Diagnoses 1976).

Gebbie, K. M., ed. *Proceedings of the Third National Conference on Classification of Nursing Diagnoses* (St. Louis: April 1978), to be published in 1980.

Source: Gordon, M. and Sweeney, M.A. *Methodological problems and issues in identifying and standardizing nursing diagnosis.* <u>Advances in Nursing Science</u>. *Vol. II, No. 1. October, 1979. p. 3. Used with permission.*

Expert nursing knowledge and judgment are essential to analyze successfully the information gathered about a patient's health and illness. Whatever the terminology (nursing diagnosis, nursing decision, problem identification), the nurse <u>must</u> make decisions for action. Assessment provides the foundation for the nursing process.

NURSING PROCESS

RESPONSE SHEET #3

Read each statement. Circle A (Agree), D (Disagree), or
? (Not sure) to indicate your response. Be prepared to explain your decisions. There are not necessarily any right
or wrong answers.

A   D   ?   1. Assessment involves both the gathering of
                     information and analysis.

A   D   ?   2. According to JCAH, initial assessments are
                     to be done on all patients.

A   D   ?   3. The use of an assessment guide provides for
                     more complete data collection.

A   D   ?   4. It is imperative that a registered nurse
                     conduct the assessment.

A   D   ?   5. Nursing diagnosis is a product of assess-
                     ment.

A   D   ?   6. A well done assessment requires many skills.

A   D   ?   7. The longer the assessment form, the better
                     the assessment.

A   D   ?   8. Assessments are done only at the time of
                     admission.

A   D   ?   9. Time does not allow for assessment of all
                     patients.

A   D   ?   10. It is most efficient to assign one nurse to
                     do all assessments.

<u>SECTION 3</u>

<u>HELP</u> WITH PLANNING PATIENT CARE

The plan of care must be documented
and should reflect current standards
of nursing practice.
                    JACH Nursing Service Standard IV

Components of Planning

To plan is "to devise a scheme for doing." It is the process
by which we think through how we will go about accomplishing
a particular task or engage in a specific endeavor. The
housewife plans what she will serve the family for dinner,
the family plans their vacation, the teacher plans learning
experiences for students and, so too, the nurse must "plan"
the care which she/he will provide patients.

Planning can be done in a variety of ways. Much planning
occurs informally. In using the nursing process, we must
document our planning activities in more formal ways. Written patient care plans, case studies, shift reports and
patient conferences are common means of formal planning.

> Written care plans for each patient are an expected
> part of nursing practice. Nursing literature de-
> scribes the purpose, value and benefits of care
> plans. In the real world of the nursing unit, how-
> ever, individual plans of care frequently are not
> developed for each patient. Why? Many reasons are
> offered, including lack of time and limited useful-
> ness. It seems time for nurses to face the issue
> realistically. Are care plans an unrealistic,
> idealized expectation? If so, why do nurses con-
> tinue to set the standard of written, individualized
> plans of care? If we value the patient as an indi-
> vidual and the nurse's responsibility for independ-
> ent (and interdependent) functioning, there must be
> a way to communicate these values. Care plans pro-
> vide the means for identifying individual patient
> needs and specifying the required nursing care
> activities.

> Care plans come in all sizes, shapes and forms.
> Often the care plan is part of the Kardex record.

Sometimes it is found on the clinical record. Far too often it is written in pencil, with sections of it left blank, then discarded when the patient is discharged. We need to make the care plan a useful and essential item. Let's begin by examining some basic facts and characteristics about care planning.

Planning, the second step of the nursing process, has three distinct components. These are:

1. Identifying patients needs/problems

2. Determining goals

3. Deciding nursing actions/activities

Identifying Needs/Problems

Identifying the patient's needs/problems is an outcome of analyzing the assessment data. A patient need can be defined as a physical or psychosocial lack or gap which results in a deficit between what is and what could or should be. Here is a list of some common areas of patient needs/problems which nursing care can help alleviate.

Common Patient Need/Problem Areas

Anxiety

Behavior

Beliefs

Bowel and Bladder Function

Comfort Level

Degree of Orientation

Depletion of Body Fluids

Family Adjustment to Illness/Impairment

Fear

Grief

Impaired Digestion

Level of Consciousness

Malnutrition

Impaired Mobility

Motor Incoordination

Pain

Impaired Skin/Integumentary Function

Relationships with Others

Loneliness

Respiratory Impairment or Distress

Ability to do Self-Care Activity

Sensory Disturbance

Sleep and Rest

Thinking Ability

Verbal Communication

Worry

(Adapted from tentative list of Nursing Diagnoses, First National Conference on Classification of Nursing Diagnosis)

Here are some "DO's" and DON'Ts" to keep in mind when discussing patient needs/problems.

<u>DO</u>

Express the need or problem as it affects the individual patient; i.e., describe the state of the patient.

Be specific enough to clearly delineate the need/problem.

Validate congruency of the needs/problems you identify.

Sources of information include the medical history and diagnosis, other health team members, the patient and family.

<u>DON'T</u>

Describe a nursing activity.

List a medical diagnosis.

Be too general.

Remember to consider possible patient problems and needs beyond those indicated by the medical diagnosis. For example, when a patient is admitted for an abdominal hysterectomy we know that the patient will need pre-op instruction, post-op relief of surgical pain, and so on. But what in addition may this individual have need for: special foods due to religious or cultural beliefs; certain comfort measures due to a previous injury? This patient may bring unique, individual needs above and beyond those resulting directly from the operation. It is essential that these needs/problems be identified.

How can we decide what needs are most important, and in what order to begin to deal with the needs or problems? One approach is to use Maslow's hierarchy of human needs for determining need priority.

MASLOW'S HIERARCHY OF NEEDS

SURVIVAL
: (*Physiological*): These are our needs for food, clothing, shelter and other things which are essential to our existence. So long as these needs go unsatisfied, the individual is little concerned with other needs and his efforts will be directed toward satisfying these basic needs.

SECURITY
: (*Safety*): Once the individual's survival needs are satisfied to at least a minimum degree, his dominant need becomes security. His efforts are directed toward satisfactions in this area. Security needs include physical safety as well as psychological safety and protection.

SOCIAL
: (*Love, affection, belonging*): When the individual has minimum satisfaction of his survival and security needs, belongingness needs become important. These include the need for love, acceptance, and approval by others—family, friends, and those he is with.

STATUS   (*Esteem, self-worth*): The individual whose survival, security and belonging-ness needs are satisfied then becomes concerned with esteem needs—for recog-nition, self-respect and self-worth.

SELF-ACTUALIZING   (*Self-fulfilling*): With the above areas of needs met at least minimally, the in-dividual's dominant need becomes self-fulfillment, becoming one's best self, using his capabilities to the fullest, seeking self-satisfaction.

(*Adapted from* Motivation and Personality, *by A. H. Maslow, 2nd Ed., Harper & Row, New York, 1970*).

<u>EXERCISE # 6</u>
From the following list check those that are well-stated patient needs/problems.

    ___ Comfort

    ___ Acute, nearly constant pain in lower back due to fall

    ___ Reddened coccxgeal area

    ___ Dehydration

    ___ Breathing difficulties

    ___ Can't sleep

    ___ Worried about returning to work

    ___ Never hospitalized before

    ___ Cholesystitis

    ___ Confused

    ___ Turn every two (2) hours

<u>Establishing Goals</u>

Once the needs/problems have been identified and priorities established, then it is necessary to determine the anticipated results. This is goal setting. Goals are like signposts along the road, routing you in a certain direction. So it is with patient care goals; they are written and used as guides to help direct your planning and care-giving activities.

How can you know when you've arrived if you don't know where you're going? In the course of patient care how often do you as the nurse ask yourself "What do I hope to achieve in my care of this patient?" Frequently? Only when you do so can you plan your nursing care to be most effective, with purposeful outcomes. Goals provide a basis for determining patient progress. They serve as criteria for evaluating the results and effects of nursing care.

<u>Characteristics of Patient Care Goals</u>

- Patient-centered

- Specific

- Measurable

- Achievable

- Time designated

- Documented (written)

A patient-centered goal is one that is stated in the context of the patient rather than the nurse. There is a tendency to describe goals in terms of what the nursing action will be rather than in the context of expected patient behavior. For example, the goal might be stated as, "to teach the patient to feed himself". That emphasizes the nursing activity— to teach—but the desired goal (result) is that the patient be able to feed himself. To say, "The patient will be able to feed himself", makes it patient-centered and better describes what the goal is. A helpful cue to assist you in developing patient-centered goals is to begin the goal statement with a preface such as:

"The patient will . . ."

or

"The patient will be able to . . ."

To be specific in goal setting means to use clear, concise and explicit terms. Examples of goals that lack specificity are "the patient will recover from his stroke" and "the patient will accept his hemiplegia". Such goals are really too broad to provide direction or to measure when the goal has been reached.

A measurable goal is one that enables us to determine that the goal has been reached. Observed patient behavior is the best indicator of goal achievement. From actions and behavior you will be able to measure to what extent there is goal attainment. Use action verbs to help describe the expected outcome—what can be observed in behavioral terms.

Attainable goals are goals that are realistic and possible of accomplishment. You must consider the patient's potential using the background of data you gathered in assessment. A variety of factors can influence the patient's attainment of goals. Consider such things as the patient's strength and endurance, knowledge and understanding, desires, courage, motivation, skills and abilities, and support system. It is important that, to the extent possible, there be patient and family involvement in the development of goals. Mutually developed goals are likely to be move realistic; the chances of attainment are greater. Consider also such resources as numbers of staff members, types of equipment, skills of the health care providers, time, and similar factors.

In setting goals a time for expected accomplishment should be specified. Sometimes we are a bit hesitant to designate a time for we fear that if, for whatever reason, the goal is not attained at the time specified then we have somehow failed. Remember that the time you specify is based upon your best judgement after considering all the facts you have at the moment. As time goes on many things change. To have a time specified with the goal, however, is very useful for it can serve as another measure for judging patient progress. Was the goal attained as specified? If not, can you identify what happened? Was the goal unrealistic? Is the patient progressing but simply at a different rate—faster? slower?

Do you now have more information that changes your ideas about the needs and goals? Were there unforeseen complications? These are the helpful types of questions that will be raised in the evaluation (fourth) phase of the nursing process if goals as described thus far are a part of planning.

As with each of the other aspects of the nursing process, it is essential that the goals be in writing and be available for use by all involved in the care of the patient.

Sometimes the question arises as to whether or not there can be goals for all patients, particularly those who are terminally ill, or chronically ill but very stable. If there is a reason for nursing care then there must be a goal. Goals for such patients may be considerably different, not reflect an expected improvement, but nonetheless be important. As an example, goals for the terminally ill patient might be such things as:

> The patient will be as comfortable as
> possible until death.
>
> The patient will have opportunity to talk
> about death.
>
> The family will learn the stages of grief
> and be able to express their feelings
> about the situation.

EXERCISE #7

Identify a patient you have recently cared for. Refer to the clinical record:

1. Review the assessment information.

2. Identify the patient's major needs/problems (those identifiable at the time of admission).

3. List the needs/problems in their order of priority.

4. Develop goals for each of the needs/problems using the six characteristics presented earlier.

The following overview can assist you in ordering needs within Maslow's hierarchy and in identifying goals related to the areas of need. This is for illustrative and reference purposes only. The needs and goals of each patient should be individualized and more specific.

OVERVIEW OF PLANNING NEEDS AND GOALS

NEEDS	GOALS
Physiological/Survival:	
Oxygen	Maintain oxygen to all cells
Food	Maintain nutrition to all cells
Sleep-rest	Achieve sleep, rest
Energy	Maintain regulating mechanisms and functioning
Body functions	
Safety/Security:	
Protection from physical harm	Prevent accidents, physical injury, deformity
Freedom from pain	Avoid infection
Predictable, orderly world	Achieve comfort
Protection from psychological distress	Achieve a therapeutic environment
Belonging/Social:	
Acceptance	Achieve productive, positive interpersonal relationships
Personal interaction	Use effective verbal and non-verbal communication
Status/Self-worth:	
Sense of value, usefulness	Participate in care and decisions affecting own health
Mastery of a skill	Learn activities for self-care
Self-actualizing:	
Increase learning	Know about cause, treatment, and/or prevention of illness
Full development of potential	Achieve optimal functioning and health

50

<u>Activities and Actions</u>

The third component of planning is to decide the specific
nursing care for the patient. The plan of care should
identify what actions and activities the nurse will engage
in. The ANA Standards of Nursing Practice state that "the
plan of nursing care includes priorities and the prescribed
nursing approaches or measures to achieve the goals derived
from the nursing diagnoses", and that "nursing actions are
planned to promote, maintain and restore the client's/
patient's well-being". The ANA practice standards also provide some criteria for these nursing actions. They include
being:

> 1. Based on scientific principles
>
> 2. Individualized
>
> 3. Considerate of a safe, therapeutic
>   environment
>
> 4. Alert to teaching/learning opportunities
>
> 5. Aware of, and using, appropriate and
>   available resources
>
> 6. Consistent with the prescribed medi-
>   cal treatment and other team members'
>   plans of care

We have all learned scientific principles and rationale in
our nursing education. To use scientific principles means
that the nursing actions reflect the knowledge and use of
sound physiological and psychosocial principles. For example,
if a patient is taking a form of digoxin, you know that it is
for the anticipated result of slowing and strengthening the
heart muscle and contraction. This physiological effect can
be assessed by checking pulse rate and volume at regularly
designated intervals. The nurse should not be dependent
upon a physician's order for direction to check the pulse,
because if the nurse is using scientific principles, he/she
knows that both the nurse and the doctor will need this
data—and so will include it as a nursing action to be
carried out.

The specific activities selected to meet the needs and attain
the goals for each patient will be varied and specific to the
individual. The activities should be directly related to the

alleviation of each identified need and related goal. It should be understood that one nursing action may contribute to more than one need, and several actions may be specified to address a particular need. Plans must show that there is a direct relationship among all of the needs, goals and nursing actions.

Providing for a safe, therapeutic environment calls for nursing activities that address both physical and psychological aspects. Raising side rails, assuring clear pathways, and providing help to ambulate may be examples of nursing actions directed toward physical safety; but consider the many nursing measures that we use to provide psychological safety and comfort. Simply our presence, particularly with a dying patient, is often therapeutic. Pre-operative instruction and other patient teaching is a good example of nursing action which helps to meet both the physical and the psychological aspects of providing a therapeutic environment.

Specific topics for patient education—such as prenatal care, instruction for the new diabetic, and pre-operative teaching—have become quite common. We must remember, however, that within the scope of nursing practice we have responsibility for patient teaching. For every patient we must ask ourselves, "What does this patient need to know?" There are few if any patients who do not have need for some teaching. Those learning needs should be indicated on the plan of care, together with the instruction (nursing actions) to be given.

In the Components of Nursing discussed in SECTION 1, coordination was identified as a major area of nursing responsibility. To coordinate we must know of available resources—persons, equipment, materials and approaches—for the benefit of patient care. It is essential that collaboration—the sharing and exchange of ideas, observations and plans—occur within the nursing staff and with other members of the healthcare team involved in the patient's care. Planning by staff members within each discipline should be compatible, enhancing that of the others. It is highly desirable for all health team members and the patient to work collaboratively in identifying one set of goals. Such goals are truly patient centered. The needs and problems identified by each discipline are merged. Then the activities and actions specific to each discipline are determined by team members within that discipline. This may appear to be idealistic, but it is a sound approach and is the current practice in many settings--especially where a problem-oriented record is in use.

The specific nursing actions and activities to be carried out will be based upon the patient's needs and goals. They will include activities specifically ordered by the physician (dependent functions), but there will also be a number of activities determined by nurses (independent functions). The following is a list of some of the most common areas of nursing action.

Major Areas for Nursing Action

Assistance needed

Beliefs, values, religion

Comfort

Communication

Doctors orders

Environmental adjustments

Hygienic care

Patient & family teaching

Prevention of complications

Problems of elimination

Problems of nutrition & fluid intake

Psychological support

Rehabilitation

Safety precautions

Referrals

Nursing activities and actions can be grouped in three major categories: doing, monitoring, teaching. Doing activities incorporate the many things that can be observed and described fairly easily. They are usually behaviors that can be actively seen, particularly those that relate to physical activities. These doing activities also include the many psychological activities the nurse engages in. These are sometimes more difficult to describe, but are nevertheless important to identify.

Monitoring actions range from gathering data about a
patient's color, vital signs and cardiac stability to noting
the patient's verbal communication and non-verbal behavior.
One might describe the nurse as *watching* with all her senses.
Monitoring activities should be specifically identified as a
part of nursing activities.

Teaching activities can range from a formal teaching program
about a particular aspect of health or illness to informal
explanations. Sometimes the patient's behavior (via questions) prompts the nurse to respond with the teaching action
of providing information on the spot. But we must also plan
to actively teach patients about their self-care, health
problems and practices, adaptations that may be needed in
habits and life style, and so on.

EXERCISE #8
     List all of the nursing activities you engage in that
     might be described as doing, monitoring, or teaching.
     Be specific as you state each activity.

DOING	MONITORING	TEACHING

Sometimes the nursing action/activity aspects of planning are referred to as "nursing orders" on the plan of care. They are just that: they are orders for nursing care. They must be taken seriously by other nurses. They should be considered as important to the nurse as medical orders. Ganong and Ganong (1980a) provide some guidelines for nursing orders. They suggest that nursing orders be:

- Easily understood

- Conscientiously carried out

- Adhered to unless the patient's condition dictates otherwise

- Respected by all nurses and staff (in the same manner that medical orders are respected)

- Taken seriously

- Challenged only with due respect for the fact that registered nurses are accountable for the plan of care and its outcomes for the patient

The significance of nursing care will be more easily recognized and valued when we are able to communicate just what nursing is. Being able to act on specific nursing orders will help to clarify what nursing is and what nurses do.

<u>Format</u>

One basic principle, however, must prevail. The plan and the orders should be set up in a format that allows it to be incorporated easily into the mainstream of activity. By this I mean that the care plan should not be something that may or may not be developed and then seldom referred to. It must be "up front". It should contain information so vital that no one dares to provide care without referring to it.

Whatever the format, three major areas of planning must be reflected on the care plan. These are as follows.

PATIENT CARE PLAN

NEEDS/PROBLEMS	GOALS	NURSING ACTIVITIES (orders)
Results of analyzing assessment data Determining priorities	Expected outcomes-results	Describes nursing action: Doing Monitoring Teaching

Here are some important items to remember in writing care plans.

RULES FOR WRITING CARE PLANS

1. Write the care plan in ink.

2. Be sure all identified problems/needs have been listed and prioritized.

3. Review assessment data before selecting nursing activities (writing the nursing orders).

4. Identify a specific goal for each problem.

5. Write the nursing activities to be done to meet each need/problem.

6. Nursing activities should be goal directed.

7. Needs, goals and activities must all be specific and individualized.

8. Update and add to care plan as new information is acquired and the patient's condition changes.

9. Discontinue nursing activities when needs have been met and problems solved.

Care plans pose a challenge to us. If used in the way described here you will find that they can assist you to:

- Individualize care

- Better organize care

- Provide continuity of care

- More easily communicate care

- Coordinate nursing care with the care provided by other disciplines

- Evaluate care

An enlightening study that examined the reasons why care plans are not written was conducted by Loucine Huckabay and Margo Neal and reported in the December, 1979 issue of Journal of Nursing Administration. Their findings indicate that success with writing care plans is multifaceted. Each of us, in whatever nursing role, must examine our practice and prepare ourselves and others to provide nursing care based upon the nursing process and utilizing effective planning as described herein.

Patient care conferences, shift reports, and informal exchange of patient information are ways available to nurses to enhance patient care planning. Such verbal methods are essential and are used regularly. They must be viewed, however, as supplemental to the core of planning carried out and documented through the patient care plan based upon the nursing process.

NURSING PROCESS

<u>RESPONSE SHEET #4</u>

Read each statement. Circle A (Agree), D (Disagree), or
? (Not sure) to indicate your response. Be prepared to explain your decisions. There are not necessarily any right
or wrong answers.

A   D   ?   1. Major components of a plan of care are
                    patient needs/problems, goals and nursing
                    activities/actions.

A   D   ?   2. JCAH requires a written plan of care for
                    each individual patient.

A   D   ?   3. Care plans should be a part of the permanent
                    clinical record.

A   D   ?   4. Maslow's hierarchy of needs is a helpful
                    guide for deciding the priority of patient
                    needs/problems.

A   D   ?   5. It is idealistic to expect that a care plan
                    will be written for every patient.

A   D   ?   6. The patient care conference is a method for
                    planning care.

A   D   ?   7. Patient care goals should be stated in
                    measurable terms.

A   D   ?   8. Observation and teaching are two important
                    areas of nursing activities to be specified
                    on the plan of care.

A   D   ?   9. The care plan should be written in pencil
                    since items change frequently.

A   D   ?   10. When possible the patient should be involved
                    in the development of the care plan.

SECTION 4

HELP WITH IMPLEMENTATION

> *It is not enough to be busy,*
> *the question is: What are*
> *we busy about?*
> Thoreau

To implement means to put into effect. This third step of the nursing process is based upon the comprehensive assessment and well-thought-out plan developed by the nurse. We consider now the content and method of implementing— providing the direct care.

Specific and unique knowledge, skill and judgement are required for delivering patient care. Formal nursing education and continuing education programs offer the major means of acquiring an essential foundation, but education alone is not enough. What additional resources are available to assist us with delivery of patient care?

Practice Guidelines

Guidelines for practice are available from multiple sources. In our examination of nursing practice in Section 1 several of these guidelines were included. The ANA Code of Ethics as well as the Standards of Nursing Practice provide general direction. Standards specific to clinical practice areas are also available. These include standards for such areas as rehabilitation, psychiatric mental health, medical-surgical, gerontology, and maternal-child nursing. Other important guidelines include the JCAH Nursing Service Standards, Medicare Conditions of Participation, and NLN Accreditation Guidelines for Community Health Nursing Services.

The nurse practice act of each state provides a legal definition and description of nursing. State boards of nursing function to uphold and implement those acts. These boards periodically issue statements and positions regarding certain nursing practices. You need to be familiar with the nurse practice act and position statements in your state. (For a summary, see HELP with Legal Aspects of Nursing Practice, by Martyann Penberth, 1979.)

State nurses associations have Councils on Practice and various other practice groups who deal with practice issues. They issue practice statements and offer assistance to nurses who have specific questions, concerns and/or problems regarding nursing practice. The Ohio Nurses Association Council on Practice, for example, has issued position statements on a variety of practice topics and concerns, as listed below.

LIST OF POSITION STATEMENTS
OF THE OHIO NURSES ASSOCIATION COUNCIL
ON PRACTICE

The Nursing Practice Role: A Statement of Belief

Patients' Rights to Nursing Care

Nursing Practice in Critical Care Units

Nursing Practice in the Operating Room

Nursing Practice in the Recovery Room

Role of the Charge Nurse

Role of Nurse Practitioners

Position Statement on the Practice of Nursing in Relation to the Physician's Assistant

Registered Nurse's Responsibility Prior to Executing Medical Orders

Guidelines for Position Description and Performance Appraisal

Role Expectations for Licensed Practical Nurses

Role Expectations for Nurses' Assistants or Aides

Position of Nurse and Pharmacist in Handling Drugs

Guidlines for Extended Pharmacy Services

Patients Bringing Medication to the Hospital

Nurse's Role in Administering Immunizations

Guidelines for Administration of Medications by School Personnel

Registered Nurse's Role in Intravenous Therapy

Role of the Nurse in the Administration of Oxytoxic Medications

Registered Nurse's Role in Performing Cardiopulmonary Resuscitation

Assistants to Nurses Performing Cardiopulmonary
Resuscitation

Registered Nurse's Role in Performing Emergency
Endotracheal Intubation

Registered Nurse's Role in Performing Endotracheal
Extubation

Registered Nurses Performing Defibrillation

Registered Nurse's Role in Removal of Arterial and
Venous Catheters

Nurse's Role in Performing Papanicolaou Smears

Other essential guidelines to the specific scope of your
practice are the nursing service policies, procedures and
standards of your own hospital or agency. Also important is
your own position description (or job performance description). You should examine these carefully and be familiar
with them.

Other valuable sources of information for guiding your nursing practice include your nursing peers and colleagues, as
well as books and journals. Become familiar and comfortable
with them and learn to use them as an ongoing source of
immediate and current help to you in the delivery of patient
care.

Caring

In statements about nursing practice, the concept of caring
appears frequently. The term is used to denote both _what_
nursing is and _how_ it is to be done. The _what_ of caring is
identified in sources as diverse as Florence Nightingale's
early list of items, and the nursing actions and activities
specified in a patient's care plan. Milton Mayeroff in an
excellent book entitled _On Caring_ addresses another aspect of
caring, one which I call the _how_ of caring. He lists eight
items as "major ingredients of caring". These are knowing,
alternating rhythms, patience, honesty, trust, humility, hope
and courage. An examination of these ingredients provides
useful insight to guide nursing practice.

Mayeroff writes, "To care for someone I must _know_
many things. I must know for example, who the
other is, what his powers and limitations are, what

his needs are and what is conducive to his growth.
I must know how to respond to his needs and what my
own powers and limitations are" (p. 13). That
powerful statement encompasses much of what we have
discussed regarding assessment and planning.

As a knowledgeable, caring nurse using the nursing process you do not care simply by force of
habit. You are open to learning and growing. You
learn from past experiences. You examine your nursing actions, determine whether you have helped or
not, and—in the light of the results—maintain or
modify your activities and actions so that you can
better help the patient. Such behavior Mayeroff
terms alternating rhythms.

Another important ingredient is patience. Mayeroff
tells us that "patience is not waiting passively
for something to happen but is a kind of participation with the other in which we give fully of ourselves. And it is misleading to understand patience simply in terms of time, for we give the
other space as well. By patiently listening to the
distraught man, by being present for him, we give
him space to think and feel" (p. 17). Here we see
our caring role with the dying patient, the patient
who is emotionally troubled, or the child who is
afraid.

An area of potential dilemma for the nurse is that
of how honest to be with patients. What do we tell
the patient with a terminal illness? How specific
should we be in sharing clinical data with patients—
such as what their BP reading is? Traditionally
nurses have communicated with the patient in vague
generalities about such matters, or even refused to
discuss it at all and simply say to the patient,
"Ask your doctor." It should be remembered that
"honesty is present in caring as something positive
and not as a matter of not doing something" (p. 18).
Remember that the patient will quickly be able to
detect the nurse who is genuine and sincere.
Actions and feelings reflect the extent of honest
caring.

About <u>trust</u> Mayeroff says, "Trusting the other is
to let go; it includes an element of risk and a
leap into the unknown, both of which take courage"
(p. 21). This is important as we allow the patient
more involvement and decision making in his care.
When we collaborate with the patient for mutual
goal setting we take a risk. We are offering the
patient greater control over the direction of his
care. In doing so we relinquish some control and
may find that the goals established are not what we
believe to be ideal or even most desirable. However, they probably will be more realistic and
possible of attainment. The patient will be more
committed by becoming actively involved in his own
care.

"The man who cares is genuinely humble in being
ready and willing to learn more about the other and
himself, and what caring involves" (p. 23).
<u>Humility</u> is demonstrated by the nurse who engages
in ongoing reassessment, revision and update of the
plan of care, and evaluation of the results of
nursing intervention. Humility means being respon-
sive and open to the patient's needs, and display-
ing pride in accomplishment.

<u>Hope</u> for the patient's progress through the nurse's
care, and the <u>courage</u> to trust that the patient will
respond to nursing care, are the bases for planning
and goal setting.

Another concept about caring is this. Before you can care
well for others you must care for yourself. This is especially important for nurses because we have seldom been
oriented to self care as a priority. We speak of self care
in the context of patient self care but give little attention
to self care of the nurse. Ann Hyde in an excellent series
of articles entitled "The Phenomenon of Caring" tells us
that "caring for ourselves and others is based on the self
care of liking, valuing and accepting ourselves. In harmony
with our own core of deepest values, we reach out to care
for each other and our world" (p. 15).

To summarize the "how" of caring, an important idea to remember is that "being with" characterizes the process of caring
itself. In caring for another person, basically we are with
him in his world in contrast to simply knowing about him from
outside.

<u>Keeping Care Current</u>

An initial care plan, however complete, is not timely indefinitely. The patient's condition changes constantly. New orders are received from the physician. Evaluation and reassessment provide updated information that dictates revisions in care planning and delivery.

The process of reassessment must include an analysis of the effectiveness of the nursing interventions up to that time. Sometimes nursing activities are carried out simply because they become routine. In nursing we have many routines, one example being a bath for every patient every day. This may be good nursing care for the majority of patients but contraindicated for the elderly, emaciated patient with dry, sensitive skin. Similarly, we may continue an activity when it no longer serves a useful purpose. For example, we may take the vital signs of hospitalized patients on a regular, frequent basis long after a normal pattern for the patient can be identified.

The nurse must also be alert to the need for additional activities of care. Has a new problem been identified? Are cues about a problem indicating an increase in severity? Is the patient exhibiting new/different behavior? It is essential that the nurse recognize and manage the changing dynamics of each patient interaction and situation. This can be a real challenge due to the magnitude of change sometimes involved. In addition, as human beings we seek comfort and in so doing risk becoming creatures of habit. This can easily engulf us in our approach to nursing care.

To keep patient care current, some questions to ask are:

1. What is the patient's response to the various
    nursing care activities?

2. Are there parts of the care plan which should
    be done more often? Less often? Discontinued?

3. Are there new activities of care which should
    be added to the plan? These may be due to such
    factors as time, patient readiness, attitude,
    changes in the patient's condition, medication
    and treatment orders, or available resources.

Continuity of Care

Continuity of care, discharge planning, referral and coordination are all items which have recently taken on increased importance. All reflect an effort to assure that patients receive appropriate care in the right setting at the right time. As increasing numbers of disciplines become involved in providing health care, coordination becomes more and more difficult. The nurse has the role of effective coordinator of patient care services. This has to be made clear for all concerned.

The concept of continuity of care is not new but it seems to be one that is difficult to incorporate in practice. For example, it is said that discharge planning should begin at the time of admission. Although discharge planning per se seldom begins that early, it is essential that it be started in sufficient time to make appropriate arrangements and notify persons to plan and provide for needed follow-up care.

For every hospitalized patient there is a potential need for follow-up care. For some the need is simply for some instruction in health routines and practices, or confirming a follow-up visit to the doctor's office or clinic. For others much more extensive planning will be required. Arrangements may need to be made with a home health care agency for care or equipment. The patient's family may need instruction, teaching, demonstrations and practice with specialized procedures and care. Do plan ahead! Poor planning or lack of appropriate arrangements can result in needless rehospitalizations for the patient.

All patients discharged from the hospital do not go directly home. Some need to be transferred to a nursing home, rehabilitation center or other specialized care facility. Here too it is essential that arrangements be made and information about the patient's care be shared with those who will be receiving the patient for care. Inform them of the patient's needs; goals already achieved; and other essential things which you know about the patient that will facilitate the transition of care.

Remember too that continuity of care is a two-way street. It is not only hospital personnel that have responsibility for discharge planning and referral. When a patient in a nursing home or home health agency is transferred to the hospital it is just as essential that a referral be sent to the hospital

in advance, with informative data about the patient. Nurses
in ambulatory settings also have an integrating role in
assuring coordination and continuity of care. Often the
patient is referred to other health and social service
agencies. The nurse often must seek out such agencies,
schedule appointments, confirm patient follow-through, and
so on. Consider what information is needed by those other
agencies as well as what reports and feedback information
would be helpful for the referring agency. The nurse in
every setting has a responsibility to coordinate patient care
with that of others in order to facilitate the patient's move-
ment through the healthcare maze. After all, no one else is
in a position to do it as well.

Much of the coordinating and referring occur verbally via
the telephone. But the most permanent, accurate and informative type of referral is the written referral. Even when the
referral is initiated by telephone, or otherwise verbally, in
nearly all instances it is essential to follow through in
writing. This serves as an accruate reference for all, and
usually provides more complete and detailed information than
what is reported verbally. It becomes a necessary part of
the patient's record.

Many agencies have developed standardized referral forms
which are interchangeable among the various community
agencies. When everyone accepts such a form, its familiarity
enhances the chances that it will be used. There is certain
essential information that most agencies need and want. Such
information usually includes demographic information about
the patient as well as a brief summary of his illness, treatment and care to date, any ongoing orders, as well as
problems/needs requiring continued attention. It is important
that the form be filled in completely.

All health team members involved in the patient's care must
be oriented to be able to contribute essential information
which will assist in assuring continuity of patient care.
Success will be only as great as the extent to which those
involved in the patient's care value the need for sharing information. Good communication is a key to good continuity
of care.

EXERCISE #9: See page 68.

NURSING PROCESS

<u>RESPONSE SHEET #5</u>

Read each statement. Circle A (Agree), D (Disagree), or
? (Not sure) to indicate your response. Be prepared to explain your decisions. There are not necessarily any right
or wrong answers.

A	D	?	1.	Better patient care is possible if a nurse uses the nursing process.
A	D	?	2.	The Nurse Practice Act of each state determines the legal scope of nursing practice in that state.
A	D	?	3.	I am familiar with my position description and the nursing service policies at the agency where I work.
A	D	?	4.	We must care about ourselves before we can truly care for others.
A	D	?	5.	Caring involves knowledge, patience, trust, and presence.
A	D	?	6.	It is important that the nurse always be honest with the patient.
A	D	?	7.	It is easier for the nurse to plan patient care according to routines rather than individualized patient needs.
A	D	?	8.	All nurses have a responsibility for assuring continuity of patient care.
A	D	?	9.	Every hospitalized patient has a potential need for follow-up care.
A	D	?	10.	Good communication is a key to good continuity of care.

EXERCISE #9

Is there an interagency referral form used
at your hospital, agency, or institution?   Yes___ No___

If so, is it used regularly for referral
and interagency exchange of information?   Yes___ No___
If not, why not?

When did you last make a patient referral?   ____________

To whom did you send the referral?   _______________________

Make a list of the departments, agencies, persons you
contact most frequently in behalf of continuity of
care for patients.

SECTION 5

<u>HELP</u> WITH EVALUATION

> *Any profession that does not*
> *monitor itself becomes a*
> *technology.*
>
> Phaneuf and Wandelt (1974)

The fourth and final step of the nursing process—evaluation —is one of challenge and change. Nurses are gaining greater skill and expertise in evaluation methodology. This has added a critically important dimension to patient care and nursing practice. The general meaning of evaluation is "to judge the worth or value of". Evaluation always requires that the judgements be made using predetermined criteria, the vari- ables that can be measured.

Within the context of the nursing process, evaluation deter- mines the quality of nursing care provided, and assesses the progress of the patient in attaining health goals. Both are major endeavors and require unique skill and expertise.

<u>Structure, Process and Outcome</u>

The Structure-Process-Outcome Model of evaluation was devel- oped by Donabedian (1966) and has been used extensively within health care.

Structure refers to the environmental resources available for providing nursing care. Such resources are human as well as material in nature. Structure factors include numbers and types of staff, fiscal and management resources, available equipment and supplies, physical environmental requirements (such as a fire alarm system), policies and procedures, and other such organizational and/or administrative matters. They are evaluated in accord with methodology that is de- signed to examine the adequacy, efficiency and/or appropriate- ness of the organization's structural framework.

The majority of early evaluation in nursing was almost exclusively structural in nature. Task analyses, bed occu- pancy and staffing studies were among the very first attempts at nursing evaluation. Today, most nursing departments are involved in very sophisticated structural evaluations. Monthly, daily, and even shift-by-shift reports and program evaluations reflect extensive use of statistical and fiscal information to examine such things as average number of hours of care per patient day based upon a patient classification system, staff utilization, program costs, policy effectiveness, and much more.

The criteria for structural evaluation are usually identified in terms of objectives, standards or conditions. Many nursing service organizations have instituted MBO Programs (Management By Objectives) that clearly identify the objectives to be used in evaluation of the nursing organization. (See HELP with Management by Objectives by Joan and Warren Ganong, 1975 for further information on this topic.)

Accreditation, licensure, certification and other approval processes conducted by voluntary and governmental bodies (such as JCAH and state health departments) focus primarily on structural aspects of evaluation. For example, of the seven JCAH Nursing Service Standards, all but one—Standard IV—relate primarily to structure.

There is an assumption that a direct, positive relationship exists between the quality of an organization's structure and the quality of patient care provided. This, however, is only an assumption. The desired quality of patient care cannot be assured simply by having an appropriate structure. Certainly structure is recognized as one important aspect to be examined. But the actual care provided and how that care is delivered (process), as well as the results of such care (outcomes), are equally important areas to be examined and evaluated.

Process evaluation examines those behaviors and activities nurses perform in delivering patient care. What specific nursing care was performed? How often? What techniques/ procedures were used? In what manner was the care provided? Such are the nature of questions to be asked in an evaluation of the process of care delivery. In essence, the major focus of process evaluation becomes what nursing care was given and how was the care delivered. Obviously there is a strong link between nursing process and process evaluation. Process evaluation provides data to determine the extent to which the nursing process was used in patient care.

Criteria for process evaluation evolve from standards of
practice which describe expected nurse performance. Nicholls
(1974) suggests that these are "means standards" because they
are nurse oriented and describe the nurse behaviors and
activities which are designed to achieve the "ends standards",
i.e., the desired changes in a patient's health status.

The focus of outcome evaluation is on results—the patient's
response to the care provided, the patient outcomes. Were
the goals attained? To what extent? Were they reached
within the projected time frame? Were the nursing actions
and activities effective? What changes in the patient's
health status occurred? Recovery rates, mortality and mor-
bidity rates, patient satisfaction, and specific clinical
data are just a few measures of patient welfare to be studied
as part of outcome evaluation.

Many persons, including Donabedian, believe that outcome
evaluation is the ultimate validator of care. It must be
realized, however, that many factors in addition to care can
influence outcomes. It is difficult at best to demonstrate
the direct cause-effect relationship between nursing care and
patient outcomes. Other variables influencing a patient's
recovery include the individual's inherent health potential,
environmental, and related social factors. Many of these
factors are difficult if not impossible to identify, control
and/or measure for their impact on patient outcome. Despite
the difficulties, much effort is being given to outcome
evaluation measures.

Table 2 provides a simple summary of evaluation in the context of the foregoing discussion.

TABLE 2

Evaluation Framework

TYPE	CRITERIA	FOCUS
Structure	Objectives	Resources: Human, Material
Process	Standards of Practice	Nursing Practice
Outcome	Goals	Patient Response

Terminology

Before we proceed further, we need to examine the terminology
of evaluation. There is much inconsistency in definition and
use. As you discuss evaluation with colleagues and examine
the literature, be sure to clarify how each term is being
used and seek to use the terms consistently yourself. The
definitions provided herewith may vary from the usage by some
other authors. Such is the state of the art at present. We
can only hope that greater familiarity and experience with
evaluation will result in greater consensus in the use of
terms.

DEFINITIONS OF EVALUATION TERMS

AUDIT:

> To examine/review for the purpose of
> verifying. (usually via records)

CRITERION:

> A specific quality, attribute, element
> which can be measured for evaluation
> purposes.

EVALUATION:

> To judge the value or worth of an item
> by the use of predetermined criteria
> for the purpose of decision-making.

GOAL: An expected/anticipated end result or
                        outcome.

MEASUREMENT: A process which provides data about the
                        extent to which criteria-standards have
                        been met. Measures can reflect quanti-
                        tative or qualitative data.

OBJECTIVE: A specific, task-oriented, behavioral
                        statement of a result to be attained.

OUTCOME: The intended, expected, desired result,
                        status or condition.

PEER REVIEW: A technique for evaluation of one's
                        performance by colleagues.

PROCESS: A way of performance (usually identified
                        in action terms).

PURPOSE: A broad description of the need for and
                        value of the intended result/outcome.

QUALITY ASSURANCE: Quality: A value judgement about what
                        constitutes a given degree of excellence.
                        Assurance: Act of making certain.

STANDARD: An agreed upon level of excellence; an
                        established norm.

STRUCTURE: The environmental framework within which
                        service is provided.

VALUES: Set of beliefs and attitudes about the
                        truth, worth, beauty of an object, be-
                        havior or thought.

Purpose of Evaluation

The term _evaluation_ sometimes has a negative connotation. For
some persons it is associated with criticism, and is seen as a
means for identifying deficiencies in one's performance or personal characteristics. Such is not the purpose of evaluation.
In fact, Stufflebeam (1971), a noted educational evaluator,
tells us that the purpose of evaluation is not to prove but to
improve. Elizabeth Hagen (in Lamonica, 1979), another noted
evaluator, agrees and states that "the primary purpose of any
evaluation is not to justify what exists; it is to provide descriptive data that will enable a person to explain the present
status and to make better decisions about what to keep or what
to change."

Examine the definition of evaluation. You will find that
evaluation involves three distinct activities—decision-
making, using criteria, and judging the value or worth of
something. In essence, there is a process occurring within
a process: i.e., evaluation is a process requiring several
sequential steps; and evaluation is a component of the nursing process.

Currently we find a great deal of emphasis in nursing and
health care on evaluation. The concept, however, is not new.
History tells us that in ancient Babylon there existed a code
of law which called for the punishment of physicians for
malpractice. Florence Nightingale was among those in the
mid-19th century to use statistical data. She compared mortality figures of the military and civilian populations
during the Crimean War, and with those she was able to up-
grade the standards of care for military personnel.

Structure-type evaluation gained prominence in the 1950's.
Process evaluation methodology developed primarily in the
1960's. Since the early 1970's greater emphasis has been
placed on outcome evaluation.

Today the trend seems to be toward the development of comprehensive evaluation programs referred to as Quality
Assurance. Quality assurance programs incorporate components
of all three types of evaluation. Schmadl's conceptual
definition of quality assurance serves to illustrate this
point.

> *Quality Assurance involves assuring the
> consumer of a specified degree of excel-
> lence through continuous measurement and
> evaluation of structural components,
> goal-directed nursing process, and/or
> consumer outcome, using pre-established
> criteria and standards and available
> norms, and followed by appropriate alter-
> ation with the purpose of improvement.*
>
> Schmadl, 1979, p. 465

The recent action by JCAH, establishing a new comprehensive
standard on quality assurance for hospitals, further confirms
this trend.

Why the recent, increased emphasis on evaluation? To some
extent it is a sign of the times. The public expects and
demands accountability. Today we deal with far more knowledgeable consumers whose approach to health care is that of
buying a service. Is the worth of the service equal to the
cost? Is the service of suitable quality? How available and
adequate is the service? Nurses must be able to provide
answers to consumer questions such as these.

The economics of health care is also a factor of major importance. As health care costs continue to soar, third party
payors (private insurance and government) as well as the individual private payor seek explanation, cost accounting, and
evidence of the value of the service. Only recently have
nurses begun to recognize and identify the worth and value of
nursing in monetary terms.

No doubt the most significant factor is the rapid advancement
of nursing and nursing practice. Licensing mandates legal
accountability, but beyond that lies the realm of professional practice. Professional practice is characterized by
autonomy. Webster defines autonomy as independence and self-
rule. Nurses today do indeed practice in a sphere of greater
independence. They possess advanced knowledge and competence.
They assume unique responsibilities in behalf of their practice. Thomas Jefferson reminds us that, "The price of freedom
is eternal vigilance." And so, as the practice of nursing
evolves to advanced levels, a posture of increased accountability is essential. Peer review, audit and the numerous
other aspects of evaluation give evidence of nursing's response to accountability.

The nurse who delivers nursing care via the nursing process
demonstrates accountability and professional nursing practice.
To use the nursing process requires that evaluation be done.

Models

There are many models of evaluation and quality assurance.
The ANA model (ANA Congress, 1975), based on the work of Norma
Lang, outlines seven sequential steps:

- Identify values.

- Identify structure, process, and outcome standards and criteria.

- Secure measurements needed to determine degree of attainment of standards and criteria.

- Make interpretations about strengths and weaknesses based on measurements.

- Identify possible courses of action.

- Choose course of action.

- Take action.

JCAH describes a six-step process. Lindeman (1976a) outlines eight steps. When these and others are examined closely, one consistently finds three major sequential activities:

Selection of criteria.

Collecting data and comparing it with the pre-determined criteria.

Taking action based upon the findings.

These are the essential components of any evaluation model. A specific model should be selected and followed when one engages in formal evaluation. It is essential that the model chosen be appropriate to the type of evaluation to be undertaken (structure, process, outcome—or some combination thereof). Selection and/or development of evaluation models is beyond the scope and intent of this manual. The following table, however, provides a helpful list with brief descriptions of many of the models which have been developed to date.

TABLE 3

SELECTED NURSING EVALUATION MODELS

Model Developer	Key Emphasis
American Nurses' Association (1973)[17]	Sets forth official standards for nursing services that are structure- or process-oriented. Not measurable in published form but provides basis for development of sub-criterion measures. The 1976 version sets forth a model for implementing standards.
American Nurses' Association (1976)[18]	
Anderson M (1973)[19]	Defines outcome criteria for patients with congestive heart failure. Suggests subclassification according to degree of physical limitation. Examples of selected criteria and rating mechanisms are included.
Aydelotte M (1973)[20]	Describes a model requiring the identification of critical time frames per type of patient problem and formulation of patient outcome criteria for each time frame.
Bidwell CM and Froeve DJ (1971)[21]	Lists an extensive set of nurse behaviors derived from Bloom's Taxonomy of Educational Objectives.
Carter J, et al (1972)[22]	Comprises a concise and definitive set of care process criteria. Provides checklists and definitions.
Commission for Administrative Services in Hospitals (CASH) (1965)	Identifies and weighs most valued nursing tasks and measures them at intervals.
Dyer ED (1967)[23]	Identifies 16 nurse traits and provides a rating scale.
H.E.W. (1974)[24]	Comprehensively lists weighted nursing process criteria with associated data gathering and statistical computation methodologies.
Iowa Lutheran Hospital (no date)[25]	Lists care process criteria for bedside audit purposes.
Joint Commission on Accreditation of Hospitals (JCAH) (1974)[26]	Recommends the development of discharge outcome criteria and critical management elements for disease-oriented diagnostic categories.
Lambertson EC (1965)[27]	Advocates theoretical framework for evaluation. Stops short of operational definitions and methodology.
Mayers M (1972)[28]	Suggests formulation of process and outcome criteria by critical time frames and by clinical or diagnostic category. Suggests data gathering methodologies but does not include specific protocols.
Medicus/Nursing Care Systems (1974)[29]	Recommends development of process and outcome criteria directly related to clinical problems or procedures and diagnostic categories. Suggests a concept of quality assurance monitoring (both retrospective and concurrent) utilizing multiple evaluative methods such as chart auditing, concurrent care review, staff/patient interviews, questionnaires, conferences, and assessment scales.
McGuire R (1968)[30]	Lists criteria for acutely and subacutely ill patients. Designed for use at bedside.
National League of Nursing (1966)[31]	Provides a self-evaluation guide to be used by a nurse to assess own functions and skills relative to patient care.
Phaneuf M (1972)[32]	Sets forth criteria relating to the seven nursing functions. Check sheets and comparative profiles are included.
Slater D, SLATER SCALE (1967)[33]	Identifies six dimensions of nurse behavior and provides rating scales.
Tate B (no date)[34]	Lists five nurse traits that may be indirectly related to quality of clinical care.
University of Michigan (SCALE)[35]	Provides categories of nursing process criteria using observation of care and physical facilities.
Veteran's Administration (1969)[36]	Measures nursing objectives. Is process-oriented.
Wandelt MA and Agar J, QUALPACS (1970)[37]	Lists 68 items on a scale. Relies upon observations and rating of care processes.
Zimmer M (1973)[38]	Recommends outcome criteria with scales to assess a range of scores per criterion. Operational evaluation tools or scales not included.

Source: Mayers, M. G., Norby, R. B., & Watson, A. B. *Quality assurance for patient care: Nursing perspectives.* New York: Appleton-Century-Crofts, 1977, p. 11. *Used with permission.*

78

EXERCISE #10
> Compare and contrast the definition of evaluation with
> the three major components of evaluation. In your own
> words describe (in words of one syllable) the three
> parts of evaluation.

1. ____

   ____

2. ____

   ____

3. ____

   ____

Criteria

The development of criteria requires time, knowledge, and
skill. It is, however, an essential endeavor. Many of the
characteristics of goals which were discussed in Section 3
are also important characteristics of criteria (specific,
measurable, and achievable). The criteria must be pertinent
to the type of evaluation being done—structure, process or
outcome.

Mayers et al. (1977, p. 17) describe criteria as "Yardsticks against
which judgements can be made . . . Criteria are descriptive
statements of performance, behavior, circumstances or clinical
status that represent a satisfactory, positive or excellent
state of affairs. Criteria describe the assessable elements
of care process or patient outcomes that can be used to
measure quality."

EXERCISE #11

In the space preceding each criterion statement place an $\underline{S}$ (Structure), $\underline{P}$ (Process), or $\underline{O}$ (Outcome) to indicate the type of criterion it is.

_____ Admission assessments are documented in the clinical record within 24 hours.

_____ Skin integrity is maintained during entire hospitalization.

_____ All patients receive pre-operative instruction within 24 hours prior to surgery.

_____ The patient will have no chest congestion 48 hours post-operatively.

_____ Performance evaluations are done annually on all nursing personnel.

_____ Nurses notes document that all post-operative patients were turned, coughed, deep-breathed q2h x 24 post op.

_____ There are written patient teaching policies.

Data Collection Methods

Data collection for evaluation purposes can be done either concurrently or retrospectively. The time of data collection is determined by the purpose of the evaluation. Concurrent collection allows for immediate appraisal of care as it is ongoing. The data source for concurrent evaluation is from "open cases"; i.e., patients who are currently receiving care.

Retrospective evaluation refers to evaluation conducted on "closed cases"; i.e., discharged patients. The purpose of retrospective evaluation is to examine patterns and trends in nursing practice and patient outcomes. Actions forthcoming from retrospective findings are reflected in changes that are generally broad in scope and systematically implemented over time.

Data can be collected via a number of different methods. Some
of the most frequently used are:

- Record Audit

- Patient Interview

- Observation

- Questionnaire

- Conference

- Reports

Clinical record audit has been, no doubt, the most common
method used for collecting both process and outcome evaluation data. This has resulted in a great deal of emphasis on
documentation. Either concurrent or retrospective evaluation
can be done via record audit. The data source is in written
form and therefore of more permanence than that of some of
the other methods, such as observation or interview. Patient
anonymity can be easily achieved using this method. That
tends to increase objectivity.

Patient interview is a method that also permits gathering
both concurrent and retrospective data. It can be done with
relative ease, and can be used to provide data for structure,
process, and/or outcome type evaluations. When gathering
process and/or outcome type data the criteria are similar to
those used in chart audits. In fact, interviews combined
with chart audit are an excellent means of increasing the
validity of findings. Patients are usually willing to participate if they are able, and assured of no risk to their care
or anonymity (when desired).

A variety of observation strategies can be used to gather
evaluation data. Rating scales and checklists help to
organize and classify the observations made relative to specific criteria. The nature of what is observed varies with
the type of evaluation. For instance, in conducting a
structure evaluation, policies, minutes and/or staffing plans
might be examined. What and how nurses practice would be the
focus of observation in a process evaluation; the patient
would be observed if outcome evaluation were the intent.
This method is used to a great extent by outside evaluators
such as those conducting a JCAH accreditation visit. It

tends not to be used as much for internal evaluations because of the element of personal discomfort associated with being observed. However, when objective criteria are used and the subjects understand the purpose their cooperation can usually be gained. It is a major strategy used for peer review and holds much potential for additional use.

Questionnaires are an appropriate and efficient means of collecting important evaluation data. Patient satisfaction questionnaires are a frequently used method of gathering certain information for evaluation of structure and/or process. Questionnaires to nursing staff can also be used to gather selected data about structure or process. Questionnaires should be designed so that the questions can be clearly understood, easily responded to, and can be completed within a reasonable amount of time. It should also be designed to facilitate categorization of the replies. Ease of return, and the subjects knowing the purpose of the questionnaire, are two factors greatly affecting the number of replies that will be received. One limitation in the use of questionnaires is the low percentage of returns usually experienced. The rate of return can be increased significantly with suitable follow-through effort.

Conferences held by staff members for the purpose of analyzing nursing practice and/or patient status can be another valuable means through which to gather process and/or outcome evaluation data. Such conferences are usually for the purpose of concurrent review. Not all patient care conferences are necessarily evaluation conferences. In an evaluation conference the pre-determined criteria are used in reviewing and interpreting the data presented. Conclusions are reached and decisions made about the actions to be taken. For example, in an outcome evaluation conference the patient goals serve as the criteria used in analyzing the data presented about the patient. Decisions can then be made about the patient's degree of attainment of the goals, any needed revisions of the goals, and the possible need for setting new goals. Conferencing is a method that holds great potential as a means of gathering valuable evaluation data—especially as nurses learn the essential skills of conducting evaluation conferences.

Report of various types contain a wealth of useful evaluation data. Incident reports, minutes of meetings of various nursing groups (i.e., head nurses), monthly statistical summaries, and shift reports are useful sources of data for

examining patterns, trends, and so on. Such reports (except
shift reports) provide retrospective type data. Reports as
an evaluation data source are used most frequently for structure type evaluation, but certain reports can also provide
data relative to process and outcome.

<u>Taking Action</u>

All evaluation efforts will be in vain if there is no action
taken as a result of the findings. What are the findings?
Is there an indicated need for changes? If so, what and how
should the changes be made?

The initial question of interest to all who participate
either directly or indirectly in the evaluation process is,
"What were the findings?" It is essential that an effective
communication network be in operation and feedback be provided. Once participants have received feedback of the
findings, their input of suggestions, ideas and/or actions
for change should be solicited. Successful implementation is
enhanced when those directly affected by the evaluation findings and potential changes are involved in this process.

The greatest risk to evaluation is failure to act. If
nothing happens once the data has been collected and examined, then passive action has been taken. Such behavior will
fail to achieve the purpose of evaluation—to improve, or at
least maintain a fully satisfactory level of performance.

Exercise #12: See page 84.

NURSING PROCESS

<u>RESPONSE SHEET #6</u>

Read each statement. Circle A (Agree), D (Disagree), or
? (Not sure) to indicate your response. Be prepared to explain your decisions. There are not necessarily any right
or wrong answers.

A   D   ?   1. The purpose of evaluation is for improve-
                     ment.

A   D   ?   2. Evaluation of structure is the most impor-
                     tant type of nursing evaluation.

A   D   ?   3. JCAH accreditation is primarily a process
                     type evaluation.

A   D   ?   4. An accurate determination of the quality
                     of nursing care can be made through a
                     clinical record audit.

A   D   ?   5. Quality Assurance programs include all three
                     types of evaluation—structure, process and
                     outcome.

A   D   ?   6. There is a comprehensive quality assurance
                     program in operation where I work.

A   D   ?   7. If there is quality in the structural com-
                     ponents of a nursing service, there will be
                     quality in patient care.

A   D   ?   8. Criteria are essential to evaluation.

A   D   ?   9. Most evaluation is done today primarily for
                     the purpose of meeting requirements and
                     regulations of outside agencies.

A   D   ?   10. Evaluation is a three-phase process.

<u>EXERCISE #12</u>

1. How familiar are you with the quality assurance
    program at your place of employment? (Circle)

    Very   Moderate   Minimal   Not at all

2. What methods do you use to evaluate your nursing
    practice?

3. What methods do you use to evaluate patient
    responses to care (outcomes)?

4. What methods are used in your agency to evaluate:

                        Structure

                        Process

                        Outcome

5. Do you regularly receive information about the
    findings of evaluations done at your place of
    employment (example: audit reports)?

                    Yes___ No___

    Then what happens?

SECTION 6

HELP WITH DOCUMENTATION

The Pen is the Tongue of the Mind
                    Cervantes in Don Quixote

Why Document?

Civilization became possible when people learned the art of
communicating ideas through the written word. Written
communications provide an element of permanence, together
with greater opportunity to examine, share, and learn.

In the healthcare industry there is an ever-increasing demand
to put it in writing. An important reason is the need for
effective coordination of the efforts of all members of the
healthcare team, as well as with the patients. And we must
be able to convey to others what nursing is and what nurses
do.

Most of us as students received instruction in charting,
especially the charting of "facts and tasks". What we
charted may have had little resemblance to what we were
learning in school about the elements of nursing care. How
many of us were taught to chart each phase of the nursing
process? The time has come when nurses, whatever their
practice setting, are no longer asked only to "chart procedures". We are expected to chart nursing care, and there
is a significant difference. In order to describe our nursing care we must be very much aware of our activities in
each of the phases of the nursing process.

Today nurses face a special challenge. We must inform all
members of the healthcare team of our role in patient care,
especially as it relates to the coordination of all services
provided to patients. Patients and families want to know,
"What am I paying for?" Nursing peers are examining and
evaluating our care in an attempt to enhance nursing as a
profession and to improve nursing practice. Patients ask,
"What are you doing for me?" A written clinical record that
reflects each phase of the nursing process provides useful

answers to all of these persons and serves as permanent legal proof of the care and service each patient receives.

Documentation of the nursing process is necessary for the following reasons:

1. To identify the nursing care given.

2. To record patients' responses and reactions to care.

3. To serve as a legal document.

4. To become a permanent record for reference.

5. To present information about the patient to all health team members.

6. To assist in coordinating patient care.

7. To systematically assemble and centralize all essential health data about a patient.

8. To serve as proof of service for the public and third party payors.

9. To provide data for determining if the nursing care met acceptable standards.

10. To help us learn better patient care.

<u>What and How to Document</u>

What should be documented? The items of a patient clinical record may be viewed as a jigsaw puzzle. When the many pieces are properly arranged, a picture emerges. A clinical record contains many forms of diverse variety and color. Much time is devoted to the design of such forms to facilitate the recording of all necessary information which might be needed and sought.

Forms and formats usually can be improved. Sometimes, however, records committees expend valuable but misguided time and energy revising record forms, and in so doing address a symptom rather than the real problem. It must be remembered that forms are only as good as the people who use them. Nurses must develop skill in their ability to document what they do. And what they do is encompassed by the nursing

process—assessing, planning, implementing and evaluating
patient care. Each of these important aspects of patient
care should be documented. Only then will the "picture" of
nursing be clearly visible.

All documentation must be as accurate, descriptive, and complete as possible. Easier said than done, but essential if
the record is to be used as one of our greatest aids in the
delivery of care. The record should contain information that
is essential and informative. It should be presented in as
concise a way as possible. It should be legible.

JCAH requirements offer guidelines for documentation:

> The nursing process (assessment, planning, imple-
> mentation, evaluation) shall be documented for
> each hospitalized patient from admission through
> discharge . . . Documentation of nursing care
> shall be pertinent and concise, and shall reflect
> the patient's status. Nursing documentation
> should address the patient's needs, problems,
> capabilities, and limitations. Nursing interven-
> tion and patient response must be noted.
>
> Nursing Services Standard IV,
> JCAH Accreditation Manual for
> Hospitals, 1980 Edition, p. 117

To avoid some of the most common errors in charting, remember
to:

- Provide detailed and adequate descriptions.

- Preface with "appears" only when you cannot validate
  the fact or incident being described.

- Use only accepted, standard abbreviations.

- Clearly differentiate inference and/or opinion from
  fact. Aim for factual data.

- Avoid information gaps and time gaps.

- Refrain from making general blanket statements (ex.,
  "Slept well.").

Skill comes with practice. So does good documentation. Old
habits and pet phrases need to be exchanged for newer formats
and more informative data. So begin now to document each
step of the nursing process in a way that will clearly show
the nursing picture.

Clinical Records

Attitudes about clinical records are also changing. In the
past the patient was seldom if ever allowed to read his
clinical record. Not so today. Often in the past, supportive healthcare personnel were denied the privilege of documenting activities and observations of patients. The clinical record was viewed primarily as a "legal document" and
seldom thought of as a vital resource to be used in planning,
providing, coordinating, and evaluating patient care.

As our concepts about the purpose and uses of the clinical
record have changed, so too has the clinical record itself
changed both in format and content. One format that has
received widespread acclaim and use is the Problem Oriented
Medical Record System, originally developed by Dr. Lawrence
Weed. The scientific principles of problem solving provide
the framework for the POMR system as they do for the nursing
process. Thus nurses using the nursing process find the
problem-oriented record system a compatible format for documenting their nursing care. It should not be concluded,
however, that one _must_ use a problem-oriented record system
in order to document the nursing process. There are many
formats and record systems that are compatible with the
nursing process. Whatever system is used must have a format
that provides for documentation of each of the four phases
of the nursing process—assessment, planning, implementation,
and evaluation.

A visit to any critical care unit will quickly confirm that
healthcare delivery is greatly enhanced by modern technology.
Superb technological capabilities exist today. But nurses
sometimes are slow to utilize newer technologies to release
us from some of the tasks, procedures and routines to which
we cling. Improved methods and systems can free us to practice the more human, caring aspects of nursing practice
which no technology can replace. Many aspects of automation
and computerization are becoming a common part of many nursing service deparment operations. It is interesting to note
that the _Journal of Nursing Administration_ has a Department

of Automation in Nursing and regularly features articles on
the topic. Both the November and December 1979 issues contain articles describing computerized clinical record systems. Not all nurses embrace technology with enthusiasm.
Weed challenges us, however, to "not feel frightened or
threatened but have the vision to reorder our loyalties and
responsibilities, learning how to embrace technology and
control it so that we can turn idealistic concern for massive
medical and social problems into constructive action."
(Weed, 1970).

The challenge is before us. The quality of our documentation
serves as a mirror reflecting the quality of our nursing care.

90

Select the clinical record for one of your recent
patients. Review it critically and answer the
following questions: (Circle the appropriate response)

1. Would a colleague (ie. nurse, therapist, physician)
    know what nursing care this patient received?

                              Yes___   No___

2. Would the nursing care be considered appropriate
    nursing practice by a peer?

                              Yes___   No___

3. If you were the patient, does the record tell you
    what the nurse did for you?

                              Yes___   No___

4. If you were paying the bill, would you pay for the
    nursing care recorded?

                              Yes___   No___

5. If the record were subpoenaed in court, would it
    reflect accurately and completely what nursing care
    the patient received?

                              Yes___   No___

6. Are all four steps of nursing process documented in
    this clinical record?

                              Yes___   No___

If not, which step(s) is/are not found?

NURSING PROCESS

RESPONSE SHEET # 7

Read each statement. Circle A (Agree), D (Disagree), or
? (Not sure) to indicate your response. Be prepared to explain your decisions. There are not necessarily any right
or wrong answers.

A   D   ?   1. The patient should be permitted to read his
                      clinical record.

A   D   ?   2. It is possible to document each step of the
                      nursing process.

A   D   ?   3. Care plans must be written.

A   D   ?   4. The care plan should become a permanent part
                      of the clinical record.

A   D   ?   5. I am familiar with the policies and pro-
                      cedures for clinical records at the agency
                      where I work.

A   D   ?   6. JCAH requires that there be written nursing
                      policies and procedures regarding confi-
                      dentiality of information.

A   D   ?   7. The use of computers is a benefit to
                      nursing.

A   D   ?   8. Nurse aides should be permitted to chart on
                      the clinical record.

A   D   ?   9. The Problem-Oriented Record System is too
                      time consuming.

A   D   ?   10. I now use a record system in which I can
                      record all steps of the nursing process.

SUMMARY

Congratulations on completing the readings and exercises in this manual. I hope that you have found this to be a worthwhile endeavor and that it has enhanced your knowledge and skill in the use of nursing process. Your patients should benefit as you use the nursing process—assessment, planning, implementation, and evaluation—to provide in your setting the care most appropriate to their specific needs and problems.

The nursing process is the keystone to excellence in nursing practice. Excellence suggests a state of quality of the highest order. John Gardner tells us that "excellence implies more than competence. It implies a striving for the highest standards". Excellence in nursing practice is our goal.

Davina J. Gosnell

ACTIONS: Nursing activities carried out in accord with the plan of care and directed toward goal attainment. Actions promote, maintain, and/or restore a patient's well being.

ANALYSIS: Examining, comparing, and contrasting information and determining its significance.

ASSESSMENT: Systematic gathering of information about a patient's health and illness and analyzing the information using nursing knowledge and judgement to determine individual patient problems and needs for nursing care. It is the first step of the nursing process.

AUDIT: Examination of records for the purpose of verifying.

CARING: Being concerned, interested, and involved with a person in such a way that human dignity and worth are valued and the commitment is toward helping the individual.

COORDINATION: To arrange many activities into an orderly pattern.

CRITERIA: Specific qualities, attributes, elements which can be measured for evaluation purposes.

CURE: Restoration of health.

DATA: Meaningful information gathered for analysis.

DOCUMENTATION: Written confirmation of any part of the nursing process.

EVALUATION: To judge the value or worth of an item by the use of predetermined criteria for the purpose of decision-making.

GOAL: An expected/anticipated end result or outcome.

IMPLEMENTATION: The doing or carrying out of nursing activities in behalf of patient care: to carry into effect the plan of care.

INTERVIEW: Verbal communication done for the purpose of soliciting specific information.

MODEL: An outlined framework by which to conceptualize a complex operation.

NEED: Physical or psychosocial lack or gap resulting in a deficit between what is and what could or should be.

NURSING PROCESS: A systematic, four step, problem-solving approach to nursing that provides for the delivery of nursing care most appropriate to the individual patient's specific needs and problems.

OBJECTIVE: A specific, task-oriented, behavioral statement of a result to be attained.

OBSERVATION: The activity of systematic and attentive watching.

OUTCOME: The intended, expected, desired result, status, or condition.

PLANNING: Formulating nursing activities in order to accomplish the goal of meeting individual patient's needs for nursing care.

PROBLEM: Resulting from a need. Used in this text synonymous with need.

PROCESS: A systematic, sequential series of actions, changes or functions that bring about a particular result.

PURPOSE: A broad description of the need for and value of the intended result/outcome.

QUALITY ASSURANCE: Making certain of the presence of a specific degree of excellence through measurement and evaluation.

STANDARD: An agreed upon level of excellence; an established norm.

STRUCTURE: The environmental framework within which service is provided.

NURSING PROCESS

A Selected Bibliography

To consult with the wisest and the greatest men; to use books rightly...If a book is worth reading, it is worth buying. No book is worth anything which is not worth much; nor is it serviceable, until it has been read, and re-read, and loved and loved again; and marked so that you can refer to the passage you want in it.

- John Ruskin -

BOOKS

Abdellah, F., et al, 1960. Patient-centered approaches to nursing. New York: Macmillan Co.

ANA Congress for Nursing Practice, 1975. A plan for implementation of the standards of nursing practice. Publ.#NP-51 7M Kansas City, MO.

In depth discussion of the standards of nursing practice. In addition, a model for implementation of quality assurance is presented. An extensive bibliography is included.

Atkinson, L., & Murray, M.E., 1960. Understanding the nursing process. New York: Macmillan Co.

Atwood, J., & Yarnall, S. R. (Eds.), 1974. Symposia on the problem-oriented record. Nursing Clinics of North America (Vol. 9, No. 2). Philadelphia: W. B. Saunders Co.

Entire volume devoted to the problem-oriented record and quality assurance.

Brodt, D., 1978. The nursing process. In N. Chaska (Ed.), The nursing profession: Views through the mist. New York: McGraw-Hill, 256-263.

Presents an overview of the nursing process including the historical background of its development. A taxonomy useful as a guide for data collection, a six-category classification of nursing practice areas for intervention, and a discussion of the parallelism of the ANA practice standards with the nursing process greatly enhance this well written chapter.

Carter, J. H., Hilliard, M., Castles, M. R., Stoll, L. D., & Cowan, A., 1976. Standards of nursing care: A guide for evaluation (2nd ed.). New York: Springer Publishing Co.

A very detailed and comprehensive description of the development of standards for an entire nursing service department. Includes many samples of forms. Explains how to develop written standards of nursing care, indices, and evaluate outcomes.

<u>Documenting patient care responsibly</u>, 1978. "Nursing Skillbook" series. Horsham, PA: Intermed Communications, Inc.

A helpful text written simply and clearly. It is filled with fine illustrations and would be a good reference for anyone seeking additional assistance with documentation.

Fromer, M. J., 1979. <u>Community health care and the nursing process</u>. St. Louis: C. V. Mosby Co.

A fine text for those in community health. Presents an overview of what's happening in the community today and the role of the nurse in it. Chapters 13 and 14 deal specifically with the nursing process and documentation.

Ganong, J. M., & Ganong, W. L.

1974. <u>HELP with the results-oriented performance evaluation program</u> (HELP #5). Chapel Hill, NC: W. L. Ganong Co.

1975a. <u>HELP with management by objectives</u> (HELP #4). Chapel Hill, NC: W. L. Ganong Co.

A "how to" manual that clearly explains the MBO concepts.

1975b. <u>HELP with the problem-oriented nursing system</u> (HELP #3). Chapel Hill, NC: W. L. Ganong Co.

A "how to" manual that clearly explains each component of a problem-oriented nursing system based on the nursing process concepts. The parts are "Understanding PONS", "Foundations", "Process", "Nursing record", "Audit", and "Education".

1978. <u>HELP with nursing audit and quality assurance</u> (HELP #2). Chapel Hill, NC: W. L. Ganong Co.

A "how to" manual that clearly explains nursing audit, standards and criteria, and the organizing of a quality assurance program.

1980a. <u>HELP with managerial leadership in nursing: 101 tremendous trifles (HELP #15)</u>. Chapel Hill, NC: W. L. Ganong Co.

1980b. <u>Nursing management</u> (2nd ed.). Germantown, MD: Aspen Systems Corp.

This fine text provides meaningful information to any nurse manager regarding the workworld of nursing, areas of nursing responsibility, and operational management. Describes the principles for a system within which the nursing process can be adopted.

Ganong, W. L., 1953. <u>The hospital scientific management project: A progress report</u>. Privately printed. Pittsburgh: Methods Engineering Council and University of Pittsburgh. See also W. L. Ganong, <u>Comparative evaluation of hospital beds</u>. Final report of research study (HEW: GN 4792). Pittsburgh: Univ. of Pittsburgh, Engineering Resource Div., Industrial Engineering Section, 1960.

Gebbie, K. M., & Lavin, M. A. (Eds.), 1975. *Proceedings of the first national conference: Classification of nursing diagnosis*. St. Louis: C. V. Mosby Co.

Harnish, Y., 1976. *Patient care guides: Practical information for public health nurses*. New York: NLN Publ. #21-1610 (League Exchange #11).

A helpful reference text for planning care. Organized in an outline form, each diagnosis or health problem includes categories of clinical manifestations, observations, plan of care, and discharge planning. Appendices and bibliography are also helpful.

Henderson, V., 1966. *The nature of nursing*. New York: Macmillan Co.

A classic nursing text which presents the author's view of nursing. She offers a definition of nursing and suggests implications for practice, research, and education.

Lamonica, E., 1979. *The nursing process: A humanistic approach*. Menlo Park, CA: Addison-Wesley Pub. Co.

A comprehensive text useful for one with a basic understanding of the nursing process. Included are selected classic articles published previously in various journals which nicely augment the writings of the author. Learning exercises follow each section.

Little, D., & Carnevali, D., 1976. *Nursing care planning* (2nd ed.). Philadelphia: J. B. Lippincott Co.

Within the context of the nursing process this text places major emphasis and focus on the components directly involved in the planning of patient care.

Mager, R., 1962. *Preparing instructional objectives*. Palo Alto, CA: Fearon Publishers.

An excellent simple text which explains clearly behavioral objectives. Although written for teachers, it is relevant to assist one in developing goals.

Marriner, A., 1979. *The nursing process: A scientific approach to nursing care* (2nd ed.). St. Louis: C. V. Mosby Co.

A very useful book for one seeking a reference text on the nursing process. An overview of each step is followed by reprints of several classic articles regarding the topic. A comprehensive, annotated bibliography accompanies each chapter.

Maslow, A. H., 1970. *Motivation and personality* (2nd ed.). New York: Harper & Row.

Mayeroff, M., 1971. <u>On caring</u>. New York: Harper & Row.

> A brief but powerful book (87 pages) which describes caring as "helping others grow". It outlines major ingredients, special aspects, meaning, and results of caring.

Mayers, M., 1978. <u>A systematic approach to the nursing care plan</u> (2nd ed.). New York: Appleton-Century-Crofts.

> Describes problem solving as a basis for care planning and expected outcomes as standards of evaluation. Various settings (hospital, education, and community) are included.

Mayers, M. G., Norby, R. B., & Watson, A. B., 1977. <u>Quality assurance for patient care: Nursing perspectives</u>. New York: Appleton-Century-Crofts.

Murray, R., & Zentner, J., 1979. <u>Nursing assessment and health promotion through the life span</u> (2nd ed.). Englewood Cliffs, NJ: Pentice Hall, Inc.

> Key physiological and psychological needs of individuals in each chronological life phase from birth to death is presented along with the role of nursing primarily in the promotion of health.

Nicholls, M. E., & Wessells, V. G., 1977. <u>Nursing standards and nursing process</u>. Wakefield, MA: Contemporary Pub. Co.

> A collection of previously published articles about nursing evaluation.

Nightingale, F., 1969. <u>Notes on nursing</u>. New York: Dover Pub. Co. (Originally published, 1860).

> A fascinating description of Nightingale's beliefs about nursing care. The relevancy of some of her remarks a century later causes one to marvel at her insight.

<u>The nursing process in practice</u>, 1974. New York: The American Journal of Nursing Co., Education Services Div. Contemporary Nursing Series.

> Compiles 36 excellent journal articles under six major sections: Overview and Development, Nurse-Client Interaction, Assessment, Evaluation, Planning Nursing Care, and Process in Practice.

Paterson, J., 1978. The tortuous way toward nursing theory. In <u>Theory Development: What, why, how?</u> New York: NLN, Publ. #15-1708.

Penberth., M., 1979. <u>HELP with legal aspects of nursing practice</u> (HELP #18). Chapel Hill, NC: W. L. Ganong Co.

> A "how to" manual that presents in an easily read, yet comprehensive style a wealth of helpful information about legal matters pertinent to nursing.

<u>Standards of nursing practice</u>, 1975. Kansas City, MO: ANA.

   Presents eight standards of care which are to guide nursing
   practice in the care of all patients.

Stufflebeam, D. L., 1971. <u>Educational evaluation and decision
   making</u>. Itasca, IL: F. E. Peacock Publishers.

   A popular text in educational evaluation that presents
   the CIPP model for program evaluation.

Yura, H., & Walsh, M. D. (Eds.), 1978a. <u>Human needs and the
   nursing process</u>. New York: Appleton-Century-Crofts.

   Presents the nursing process as the core process for the
   practice of nursing, and basic human needs as the terri-
   tory of nursing. Two levels are pursued: the healthy
   person and how to ensure health maintenance, preservation,
   and prevention of illness; and human need violation. Con-
   tributing authors expand upon these two levels using the
   nursing process as the framework.

Yura, H., & Walsh, M. B., 1978b. <u>The nursing process: Assessment,
   planning, implementing, evaluating</u> (3rd ed.). New York:
   Appleton-Century-Crofts.

   Develops the problem-solving method as a basis for the
   nursing process. Discusses each component of the nursing
   process and its application. Also presents the historical
   background, framework, and future of the nursing process.

ARTICLES

Block, D., 1974. Some crucial terms in nursing: What do they
   really mean? <u>Nursing Outlook</u>, <u>22</u> (10), 689-694.

Chinn, P. (Ed.)

   1979. Nursing diagnosis. <u>Advances in Nursing Science</u>, <u>2</u> (1)

   1980. Nursing intervention. <u>Advances in Nursing Science</u>,
   <u>2</u> (2).

   Entire issues devoted to topics as indicated.

Donebedian, A., 1966. Evaluating the quality of medical care.
   <u>MMFQ/Health and Society</u>, <u>64</u> (July), 166-206.

   Presents the structure-process-outcome model for evaluation.
   Discusses application to the health care setting with focus
   specifically on medical care.

Eggland, E. T., 1980. Charting: How and why to document your
   care daily—and fully. <u>Nursing 80</u>, <u>10</u> (2), 38-43.

   Provides specific examples of pertinent daily nurses' notes;
   includes how to describe signs and symptoms, and do's and
   don'ts of daily charting. Helpful and practical.

Fehlau, M. T., 1975. Applying the nursing process to patient care in the operating room. Nursing Clinics of North America (Vol. 10, No. 4), 617-623.

Illustrates the usefulness of the nursing process in providing patient care to the surgical patient including during the time in the operating room. A sample case study illustrates.

Fuller, D., & Rosenaur, J., 1974. A patient assessment guide. Nursing Outlook, 22 (7), 460-462.

Presents a nursing assessment tool developed for use with ambulatory patients in a primary health care setting.

Gane, D., 1973. Sparky: A success story. AJN, 73 (7), 1176-1177.

Cleverly illustrates by use of a case study about a dog, how to document each step of the nursing process using POR.

Ganong, J. M., & Ganong, W. L., 1977. The head nurse as hospital integrator. Supervisor Nurse, 8 (3), 27-39.

Gluck, J., 1979. The computerized medical record system: Meeting the challenge for nursing. Journal of Nursing Administration, 9 (12), 17-24.

A system of computerized records in an HMO is described. The author notes that such a change increased nursing's accountability and responsibility for complete, consistant documentation. She notes that nurses must be comfortable with patient assessment, patient management, and documentation in order to effectively utilize the system.

Gordon, M., 1976. Nursing diagnosis and the diagnostic process. AJN, 76 (8), 1298-1300

Discusses the term nursing diagnosis and describes its use in the nursing process.

Gosnell, D. J., 1973. An assessment tool to identify pressure sores. Nursing Research, 22 (1), 55-59.

Describes the use of an assessment tool developed specifically to identify patients most prone to develop pressure sores.

Hays, J., 1966. Analysis of nurse-patient conversations. Nursing Outlook, 14 (9), 32-35.

A study of 100 nurse-patient conversations identifies some major communication problems and suggests some appropriate responses.

Henderson, V., 1973. On nursing care plans and their history. Nursing Outlook, 21 (6), 378-379.

Describes the early origin of nursing care plans.

Hofling, A. L., McGugin, M. D., & Merkel, S. I., 1979. The
    importance of maintenance in implementing change: An ex-
    perience with problem oriented recording. Journal of
    Nursing Administration, 9 (12), 43-48.

    Describes the activities that must be ongoing in order to
    maintain the level of quality desired after instituting a
    major change such as the introduction of POR. Skill rein-
    forcement, audit, climate, feedback of management, and
    peer support were all found to be important factors.

Huckabay, L. M. D., & Neal, M. C., 1979.· The nursing care plan
    problem. Journal of Nursing Administration, 9 (12), 36-42.

    Describes a study of the reasons why care plans generally
    are not written. Findings suggest that positive reinforce-
    ment, more knowledge about care planning, and the nurse's
    value of care plans were all important factors in the extent
    to which care plans were written.

Hyde, A., 1976/1978. The phenomenon of caring. American Nurses
    Foundation - Nursing Research Report, 10 (3) and 12 (2).

    Presents a 6-part series on caring. Causes one to do some
    value examining and self assessment of beliefs. Stimulating
    and well written.

Lewis, L., 1968. This I believe...about nursing process, key to
    care. Nursing Outlook, 16 (5), 26-29.

    A clear explanation of the nursing process and its use.

Lindeman, C., 1976a. Measuring quality of nursing care, part I.
    Journal of Nursing Administration, 6 (6), 7-11.

Lindeman, C., 1976b. Measuring quality of nursing care, part two.
    Journal of Nursing Administration, 6 (9), 5-8.

    Offers an overview of an 8-step evaluation model and discusses
    issues related to measuring the quality of nursing care.

McCain, F., 1965. Nursing by assessment— not intuition. AJN,
    65 (4), 82-84.

    Describes the development of an assessment guide and lists
    the assessment factors included.

McCloskey, J. D., 1980. Nurses' orders: The next professional
    breakthrough? RN, 43 (2), 99-113.

    Emphasizes that assessment by the nurse leads to a nursing
    diagnosis—which pinpoints what nursing is and what nursing
    does. Nursing diagnosis presented as a symbol of the nursing
    profession's new independence, accountability, and potential
    influence on the health care scene. Includes the entire
    nursing process, and suggests ways to close the gap between
    nursing education and nursing practice.

102

McNeill, D. G., 1979. Developing the complete computer-based information system. <u>Journal of Nursing Administration</u>, <u>9</u> (11), 34-46.

Describes the PROMIS (Computerized Problem-Oriented Medical Information System). Presents an overview of the system and describes its use at the Medical Center Hospital of Vermont.

McPhetridge, L. M., 1968. Nursing history: One means to personalize care. <u>AJN</u>, <u>68</u> (1), 68-75.

Presents an extensive nursing history format and describes its use.

Nicholls, M. E., 1974. Quality control in patient care. <u>AJN</u>, 74 (3), 456-459.

Provides a clear discussion of the components of a quality assurance program. Relates it within the nursing process framework.

Phaneuf, M., 1966. The nursing audit for evaluation of patient care. <u>Nursing Outlook</u>, <u>14</u> (6), 51-54.

Presents a tool for audit of clinical records.

Phaneuf, M. C., & Wandelt, M. A., 1974. Quality assurance in nursing. <u>Nursing Forum</u>, <u>13</u> (4), 328-345.

Six characteristics of a quality assurance program are suggested and three methods/instruments for measuring the quality of nursing care are discussed.

Schmadl, J. C., 1979. Quality assurance: Examination of the concept. <u>Nursing Outlook</u>, <u>27</u> (7), 462-465.

An indepth look at the meaning and implications of quality assurance.

Sculco, C. D., 1978. Development of a taxonomy for the nursing process. <u>Journal of Nursing Education</u>, <u>18</u> (6), 40-48.

Provides a taxonomy for the nursing process. Useful for planning and evaluating care as well as performance by the care giver.

Smith, D., 1971. Writing objectives as nursing practice. <u>AJN</u>, <u>71</u> (2), 319-320.

Presents a clear and concise approach to the development of patient-centered goals.

Stevens, B. J., 1972. Why won't nurses write nursing care plans? <u>Journal of Nursing Administration</u>, <u>2</u> (6), 6-7, 91-92.

Describes some of the fallacies and errors in our attempts to develop meaningful, useful care plans. Suggests corrective steps to take so that care plans will be written.

Vasey, E., 1979. Writing your patient's care plan...effectively.
    Nursing '79, 9 (4), 67-71.

    Provides guidelines for developing useful written care plans.

Wagner, B., 1969. Care plans: Right, reasonable, and reachable.
    AJN, 69 (5), 986-990.

    Explains the characteristics of good care plans and how to
    use them.

Weed, L. S., 1970. Technology is a link, not a barrier for doc-
    tor and patient. Modern Hospital, 114 (2), 80-83.

    Presents the positive benefits which technology provides to
    enhance the delivery of patient care.

Wolff, H., & Erickson, R., 1977. The assessment man. Nursing
    Outlook, 25 (2), 103-107.

    Provides an easy-to-use tool for head-to-toe assessment.
    Assists one to organize data rapidly and logically.

Woody, M., & Mallison, M., 1973. The problem oriented system
    for patient centered care. AJN, 73 (7), 1168-1175.

    Describes how to document each step of the nursing process
    using POR. Helpful illustrations.

Zimmerman, D., & Gohrke, C., 1970. The goal directed nursing
    approach: It does work. AJN, 70 (2), 306-310.

    Presents a case study showing effective use of goals to
    guide nursing care.

ADDENDUM TO BIBLIOGRAPHY

The Patient Assessment Series. New York: American Journal of
    Nursing Company, Educational Services Division,

    Eighteen units on basic aspects of patient assessment
    prepared by experts in consultation with clinical nurse
    specialists and American Journal of Nursing editors.

SELF-ADMINISTERED POST-TEST   105

Instructions: Please list what you <u>know</u> and how you <u>feel</u> about this subject (after completing your study program). Include as many items as possible, briefly and frankly. Use other side if necessary.

FACTS (Cognitive Information): What I <u>Know</u> About This Subject	FEELINGS (Affective Information): How I <u>Feel</u> About This Subject
	Identify your feelings about each fact.

FACTS (Cognitive Information): What I Know About This Subject:

1.
2.
3.
4.
5.
6.
7.
8.
9.
10.

FEELINGS (Affective Information): How I Feel About This Subject:

1.
2.
3.
4.
5.
6.
7.
8.
9.
10.

Some Feelings

Agitated
Amused
Angry
Anxious
Apprehensive
Belittled
Bemused
Bewildered
Confused
Content
Depressed
Disaffected
Excited
Expectant
Faint
Foolish
Glad
Happy
Hurt
Impressed
Inspired
Irritated
Joyful
Kindly
Lost
Morose
Numb
Optimistic
Proud
Provoked
Puzzled
Queer
Querulous
Relieved
Sorrowful
Stunned
Thrilled
Upset
Wondering

NAME ________________________   TITLE ________________________   DATE ____________

AGENCY ______________________   CITY & ZIP ___________________________

SELF-EVALUATION

You were invited to add your personal objectives. How well have you met these objectives? Please indicate your feelings about your degree of achievement by checking one column for each objective. (If you are score-minded, you may total your number of check marks in each column and compute your total score.)

I ACHIEVED OBJECTIVE: (Check one column/objective)				OBJECTIVES
Very well	Quite well	Fairly	Poorly	Upon completion of study program I can:
				1. *Explain each step of the nursing process.*
				2. *Conduct nursing assessments.*
				3. *Develop comprehensive patient care plans.*
				4. *Implement nursing care based upon assessment and planning.*
				5. *Identify and utilize evaluation techniques to determine the adequacy, appropriateness, efficiency, and effectiveness of nursing care provided.*
				6. *Document each step of the nursing process.*
				7. *My personal objectives:*
4x __ = __	3x __ = __	2x __ = __	1x __ = __	Total Score: _______________

COMMENTS:

OVER

PROGRAM EVALUATION

RESPONSE SHEET

INSTRUCTIONS: *Please evaluate each of the following items as it relates to this program. For each item, check the column that best expresses your opinion.*

		Really OK	*Just* OK	*Not* OK
A.	**Subject Content**			
	1. Related to Objectives	—	—	—
	2. Clearly Presented	—	—	—
	3. Comprehensive	—	—	—
	4. Helpful to Me	—	—	—
	5. Interesting	—	—	—
	6. New Information	—	—	—
B.	**Involvement** (Exercises)			
	1. Helped with Learning	—	—	—
	2. Relevant	—	—	—
	3. Stimulating	—	—	—
	4. Truly *Felt*	—	—	—
C.	**Leader** (Presentation Methods)			
	1. Enjoyable	—	—	—
	2. Organized	—	—	—
	3. Helpful	—	—	—
	4. Respectful	—	—	—
	5. Stimulating	—	—	—
	6. Empathetic	—	—	—

OTHER EVALUATIVE COMMENTS AND SUGGESTIONS:

ORDER FORM FOR HELP MANUALS AND TRAINING AIDS
by
Joan Ganong, RN, MS and Warren Ganong, CMC
and our Nurse Consultant Associates

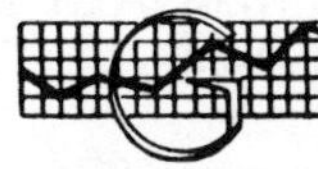

*The **HELP** Series of Management Guides and Workbooks contains, from 64 to 152 pages each, 8½"x11" in size, soft cover for ease of use, with discussion sheets at the end of each section. Our workshops, using these manuals, have been approved throughout the USA for CEU credit from universities, technical institutes, state nurses associations and licensing agencies. **Quantity Discounts:** 8% on 6-10 copies, 15% on 11-20, 22% on 21 and over. Shipping and handling costs are in addition except when payment accompanies your order.*

HELP NO.	TITLE	PUBL. DATE	LIST PRICE (1-5 copies)	NUMBER ORDERED
# 1	**HELP for the Head Nurse:** A Management Guide (3rd Edition) . . . *Our time-tested best seller. Basic guide for the modern nurse manager as effective patient care integrator. A valued orientation/promotion gift. 88 pp.*	'78	$ 9.50	__________
# 2	**HELP with Nursing Audit & Quality Assurance** (3rd Edition). . . *Assists in meeting accreditation requirements; used widely by AQP and audit committees. Helps with the human and technical modes in implementing the audit procedure. 114 pp.*	'78	10.75	__________
# 3	**HELP with the Problem-Oriented Nursing System** (PONS). . . *An integrated view of the nursing process as a management technique; problem-oriented charting, with or without a problem-oriented medical record (POMR). 108 pp.*	'75	10.50	__________
# 4	**HELP with Management by Objectives** (MBO). . . *Applying management by objectives to personnel management and to patient care management. Step-by-step instructions for the goal-oriented approach in unit management (NMBO), direct patient care (NBO), and the service-minded management of other agency departments. 132 pp.*	'75	11.75	__________
# 5	**HELP with the Results-Oriented Performance Evaluation Program** (ROPEP) . . . *Implementation guidelines for an effective personnel self-evaluation technique. Researched, introduced and agency-tested as a potent, viable alternative to traditional personnel appraisal procedures. Helps you meet JCAH 1980 standards for performance appraisal. 101 pp.*	'74	10.50	__________
# 6	**HELP with Career Ladders in Nursing** . . . *Cost-effective, in-house career planning: clinical, mgt., educational and research tracks. Expanding career options at all levels through agency-developed criteria for meeting performance requirements; including length of service, salary, EEO, labor relations and budgetary considerations. 142 pp.*	'77	13.75	__________
# 7	**HELP with Annual Budgetary Planning and Control** (ABP) . . . *Proven techniques for responsible involvement. Achieving financial and patient care accountability through Program Performance Planning and MBO. Cost control methods. 90 pp.*	'76	9.75	__________
# 8	**HELP with Innovative Teaching Techniques** (ITT) (2nd Edition) . . . *Modern techniques in affective education. The thinking and feeling components of the learning process. Application to patient teaching, inservice and continuing education. 152 pp.*	'76	13.95	__________
# 9	**HELP for Hospital Department Heads:** A Management Guide . . . *Management functions, techniques and skills for securing service-oriented, cost-controlled results in meeting agency goals. The human and technical modes in department leadership. 84 pp.*	'76	9.50	__________
#10	**HELP with Motivational Management** . . . *Positive methods of getting results and avoiding grievances. Leadership practices and motivational methods in union and non-union agencies. 92 pp.*	'76	9.95	__________
#11	**HELP for the LPN:** The Leadership Role . . . *Becoming more effective as an LPN/LVN team leader and charge nurse. Leadership styles, skills and techniques. For LPN's/LVN's who are in, or aspire to, leadership roles and a career development program. 71 pp.*	'75	8.25	__________
#12	**HELP for the Unit Secretary:** The Service Coordinator Concept . . . *The unit secretary's role on the patient care team. Skills, techniques, challenges and opportunities. Developing the helping relationship. 64 pp.*	'75	8.25	__________
#13	**HELP with Primary Nursing:** Accountability through the Nursing Process . . . *Implementation guidelines for a forward-looking alternative method for the delivery of goal-oriented patient care. Use of process-oriented concepts; staffing, costs, benefits; practical application of the nursing process. 90 pp.*	'77	9.75	__________
#14	**HELP with Student Clinical Performance Evaluation** . . . *An effective results-oriented plan for evaluating student clinical performance using pre-set standards. Combines learning contracts with mutually-developed objectives, building on assets and student self-evaluation. 90 pp.*	'77	9.75	__________
#15	**HELP with Managerial Leadership in Nursing:** 101 Tremendous Trifles . . . *This is an update of our unique, practical collection of management mini-guides from the HELP Series. A copious compendium of nursing management concepts, tips, skills, techniques; "the best of its kind," a "workshop gem." 160 pp.*	'80	12.50	__________
#16	**101 Exciting Exercises:** HELP Worksheets for Nurse Managers and Educators . . . *Companion to #15. These help make life easier for the nurse educator/manager. 109 pp.*	'78	10.95	__________
#17	**HELP with Career Planning:** A Workbook for Nurses , *by Cecelia Golightly, RN, MPH* . . . *Helps **every** nurse (student, staff, manager) plan own goals, growth, finances; a real winner. 95 pp.*	'79	9.75	__________
#18	**HELP with Legal Aspects of Nursing Practice,** *by Martyann Penberth, RN, MS, MPH.* . . . *Practical study guide and reference handbook: state practice acts, liability, concepts, issues. 116 pp.*	'79	10.50	__________
#19	**HELP with the Nursing Process,** *by Davina J. Gosnell, RN, PhD.* . . . *Timely, topical, practical, thorough, easy-to-use guide to the nursing process. Will help nurses at all levels (students, practitioners, managers) apply JCAH 1980 standards. 110pp.*	'80	10.95	__________

NURSING MANAGEMENT (2nd Edition): (See over; check here for autographed copies _____) 477 pp . . . ASPEN   '80   19.95   __________

CASES IN NURSING MANAGEMENT: (See over; check here for autographed copies________) 372pp. . . ASPEN   '79   19.95   __________

SUBSCRIPTION to G-GRAM, Newsletter (for Nurse Managers & Educators), *plus* Pocket Planner/Diary, Annual   Sub. . . . .   11.95   __________

SEND MORE INFO. ON: Consulting ☐   In-house Workshops ☐   Nursing Management Seminar ☐   Area Workshops ☐

NAME OF AGENCY _________________________________TEL. NO._________DATE_______

ADDRESS ___________________________CITY_______________STATE_________ZIP_________

SIGNED _____________________________ TITLE_________________________   (over)

8/80

Please Reply To: W.L. Ganong Company   •   Homestead House   •   P.O. Box 2727, Chapel Hill, NC 27514   •   919/929-0421